v

Preface

The intelligence community (IC) faces voluminous amounts of scientific information produced and available on a global scale. To improve analysis of the information, the Technology Warning Division (TWD) of the Defense Intelligence Agency's (DIA's) Defense Warning Office (DWO) asked the National Research Council (NRC), in 2004, to establish the Committee on Defense Intelligence Agency Technology Forecasts and Reviews. That committee authored the report *Avoiding Surprise in an Era of Global Technology Advances.*[1] *Avoiding Surprise* provided the IC with a technology warning methodology not previously available to it and led the DIA to request that the NRC establish a standing committee to continue to provide related assistance. In May 2005, the Standing Committee for Technology Insight—Gauge, Evaluate, and Review (TIGER) was established to assist the DWO of DIA in formulating future studies to be completed by NRC ad hoc committees. This report of the ad hoc Committee on Military and Intelligence Methodology for Emergent Neurophysiological and Cognitive/Neural Science Research in the Next Two Decades is the third report to be produced under the purview of the TIGER Standing Committee.[2]

We wish to express our sincere appreciation to the committee members, the staff of the DWO/TWD and their IC partners for their sponsorship and active participation, and Angelique Reitsma of the University of Pennsylvania. We also

---

[1]National Research Council. 2005. *Avoiding Surprise in an Era of Global Technology Advances.* Washington, D.C.: The National Academies Press. Available from http://www.nap.edu/catalog.php?record_id=11286.

[2]The previous reports in the series were *Critical Technology Accessibility* (2006) and *Nanophotonics: Accessibility and Applicability* (2008), both published by the National Academies Press, Washington, D.C.

appreciate the contribution of the staff of the TIGER Standing Committee led by Mike Clarke and the staff of the Board on Behavioral, Cognitive, and Sensory Sciences led by Chris Hartel.

Christopher C. (Kit) Green, *Chair*
Diane E. Griffin, *Vice Chair*
Committee on Military and Intelligence Methodology for
    Emergent Neurophysiological and Cognitive/Neural
    Science Research in the Next Two Decades

Acknowledgment of Reviewers

This report has been reviewed in draft form by individuals chosen for their diverse perspectives and technical expertise, in accordance with procedures approved by the National Research Council's (NRC's) Report Review Committee. The purpose of this independent review is to provide candid and critical comments that will assist the institution in making its published report as sound as possible and to ensure that the report meets institutional standards for objectivity, evidence, and responsiveness to the study charge. The review comments and draft manuscript remain confidential to protect the integrity of the deliberative process. We wish to thank the following individuals for their review of this report:

Floyd Bloom (NAS, IOM), The Scripps Research Institute,
Ruth David (NAE), ANSER, Inc.,
Robert Desimone (NAE), Massachusetts Institute of Technology,
David Dinges, University of Pennsylvania School of Medicine,
Stephen Drew (NAE), Drew Solutions LLC,
Michelle Gelfand, University of Maryland,
Gilbert Omenn (IOM), University of Michigan Medical School,
Richard Pew, BBN Technologies,
Mark Rise, Medtronic, Inc.,
Richard Thompson (NAS), University of Southern California, and
Charles Wilson (IOM), HealthTech.

Although the reviewers listed above have provided many constructive comments and suggestions, they were not asked to endorse the conclusions or recommendations nor did they see the final draft of the report before its release. The review of this report was overseen by John Bailar (IOM), University of Chicago (emeritus), and Richard Davidson, University of Wisconsin, Madison. Appointed by the NRC, they were responsible for making certain that an independent examination of this report was carried out in accordance with institutional procedures and that all review comments were carefully considered. Responsibility for the final content of this report rests entirely with the authoring committee and the institution.

Contents

5 POTENTIAL INTELLIGENCE AND MILITARY APPLICATIONS OF
   COGNITIVE NEUROSCIENCE AND RELATED TECHNOLOGIES   124
   Introduction, 124
   Market Drivers of Cognitive Neuroscience and Related Technologies as
        Indicators of the Demand for COTS Technologies, 127
      Overview, 127
      The Search for New and Patentable Neurophysiological Agents, 129
      Market Barriers and How the Drivers May Change, 130
   Technology Assessments: Neuropsychopharmacology, 134
   Technology Assessments: Distributed Human-Machine Systems and
        Computational Biology, 140
   Findings and Recommendation, 141
   References, 144

APPENDIXES

Acronyms

ABC	ATP-binding cassette
ACh	acetylcholine
AugCog	augmented cognition
BBB	blood-brain barrier
BCI	brain–computer interface
BMI	brain–machine interface
BOLD	blood-oxygenation-level-dependent
CBF	cerebral blood flow
CIA	Central Intelligence Agency
CIOMS	Council for International Organizations of Medical Sciences
CNS	central nervous system
COM	cultural orientation model
COTS	commercial off-the-shelf (technology)
CT	computed tomography
CW	continuous wave
DEPS	Division on Engineering and Physical Sciences
DHMS	distributed Human-Machine system
DIA	Defense Intelligence Agency
DOD	Department of Defense
DoH	Declaration of Helsinki
DWO	Defense Warning Office

EAP	electroactive polymer
EEG	electroencephalography
EFGCP	European Forum for Good Clinical Practice
EMG	electromyography
ERP	event-related potential
FDA	Food and Drug Administration
fMRI	functional magnetic resonance imaging
fNIR	functional near-infrared spectroscopic imaging
fTDS	functional transcranial Doppler sonography
GABA	gamma aminobutyric acid
HPC	high-performance computing
HSCB	human, social, cultural, and behavioral
HTS	Human Terrain System
HTT	Human Terrain Team
IC	intelligence community
ICH	International Conference on Harmonization
IED	improvised explosive device
IQ	intelligence quotient
IR	infrared
IRB	institutional review board
LED	light-emitting diode
LSD	lysergic acid diethylamide
MAO	monoamine oxidase
MEG	magnetoencephalography
MOHME	Ministry of Health and Medical Education
MPTP	1-methyl-4-phenyl-1,2,3,6-tetrahydropyridine
MR	magnetic resonance
MRI	magnetic resonance imaging
MRS	magnetic resonance spectroscopy
NATO	North Atlantic Treaty Organization
NIH CATIE	National Institutes of Health Clinical Antipsychotic Trials of Intervention Effectiveness
NIMH	National Institute of Mental Health
NIRS	near-infrared spectroscopy
NIRSI	near-infrared spectroscopy imaging
NLP	neuro-linguistic programming

NRC	National Research Council
PET	positron emission tomography
PLA	People's Liberation Army
POW	prisoner of war
PTSD	post-traumatic stress disorder
QEEG	quantitative electroencephalography
RNA	ribonucleic acid
SCP	slow cortical potential
SMR	sensorimotor rhythm
SQUID	superconducting quantum interference device
S&T	science and technology
tCDS	transcranial direct current stimulation system
THC	tetrahydrocannabinol
TIGER	(Standing Committee on) Technology Insight—Gauge, Evaluate and Review
TWD	Technology Warning Division
UN	United Nations
UNESCO	United Nations Educational, Scientific and Cultural Organization
WMA	World Medical Association

Summary

CONTEXT

The intelligence community (IC) faces the challenging task of analyzing extremely large amounts of information on cognitive neuroscience and neurotechnology, deciding which of that information has national security implications, and then assigning priorities for decision makers.[1] It is also challenged to keep pace with rapid scientific advances that can only be understood through close and continuing collaboration with experts from the scientific community, from the corporate world, and from academia. The situation will become more complex as the volume of information continues to grow. The Committee on Military and Intelligence Methodology for Emergent Neurophysiological and Cognitive/Neural Science Research in the Next Two Decades was tasked by the Technology Warning Division of the Defense Intelligence Agency's (DIA's) Defense Warning Office to identify areas of cognitive neuroscience and related technologies that will develop over the next two decades and that could have military applications that might also be of interest to the IC. Specifically, the DIA asked the National Research Council (NRC) to perform the following tasks:

• Review the current state of today's work in neurophysiology and cognitive/ neural science, select the manners in which this work could be of interest to

---

[1]The intelligence community is made up of approximately 16 entities across the executive branch. A detailed listing of all IC members is found on the United States Intelligence Community Web site at http://www.intelligence.gov/1-members.shtml. Last accessed on March 17, 2008.

1

national security professionals, and trends for future warfighting applications that may warrant continued analysis and tracking by the intelligence community,[2]

• Use the technology warning methodology developed in the 2005 National Research Council report *Avoiding Surprise in an Era of Global Technology Advances* (NRC, 2005) to assess the health, rate of development, and degree of innovation in the neurophysiology and cognitive/neural science research areas of interest, and

• Amplify the technology warning methodology to illustrate the ways in which neurophysiological and cognitive/neural research conducted in selected countries may affect committee assessments.

The label "cognitive" in the title and elsewhere in this report is used in a broad sense, unless specifically noted otherwise in the report itself, to refer to psychological and physiological processes underlying human information processing, emotion, motivation, social influence, and development. Hence, it includes contributions from behavioral and social science disciplines as well as contributing disciplines such as philosophy, mathematics, computer science, and linguistics. The label "neuroscience" is also used in a broad sense (unless specified otherwise) and includes the study of the central nervous system (e.g., brain) and somatic, autonomic, and neuroendocrine processes.

This summary includes the committee's key findings and recommendations, numbered to facilitate access to related text in Chapters 2-5, which also include additional findings.

THE BOTTOM LINE

Cognitive neuroscience and its related technologies are advancing rapidly, but the IC has only a small number of intelligence analysts with the scientific competence needed to fully grasp the significance of the advances. Not only is the pace of progress swift and interest in research high around the world, but the advances are also spreading to new areas of research, including computational biology and distributed Human-Machine systems with potential for military and intelligence applications. Cognitive neuroscience and neurotechnology constitute a multifaceted discipline that is flourishing on many fronts. Important research is taking place in detection of deception, neuropsychopharmacology, functional neuroimaging, computational biology, and distributed human-machine systems, among other areas. Accompanying this research are the ethical and cultural implications and considerations that will continue to emerge and will require serious thought and actions. The IC also confronts massive amounts of pseudoscientific

---

[2]In negotiation with the sponsor on the statement of task, this item was intentionally left broad in scope to allow the committee to select the areas within the field of cognitive neuroscience that it believed should be of interest to the intelligence community. The selected areas of interest are discussed in Chapters 2 through 4.

information and journalistic oversimplification related to cognitive neuroscience. Further, important research outside the United States in cognitive neuroscience is only just beginning, making it almost impossible to attempt to accurately assess the research at this point in time.

Key Finding (Finding 5-5). The recommendations in this report to improve technology warning for cognitive neuroscience and related technologies are unlikely to succeed unless the following issues are addressed:

- Emphasizing science and technology as a priority for intelligence collection and analysis.
- Appointing and retaining accomplished IC professionals with advanced scientific and technical training to aid in the development of S&T collection strategies.
- Increasing external collaboration by the IC with the academic community. It should be noted that some components of the IC have made great strides in reaching out to the academic community.

Key Recommendation (Recommendation 5-1). The intelligence community should use a more centralized indication and warning process that involves analysis, requirement generation, and reporting. Engagement with the academic community is required and is good, but it is not now systematically targeted against foreign research.

Challenges to the Detection of Psychological States and Intentions via Neurophysiological Activity

Great progress has been made over the last quarter century, particularly the last 10 to 15 years, in understanding the physiological and neural bases of psychological processes and behavior. More progress is expected as more sophisticated biopsychosocial theoretical models are developed and tested using ever more sophisticated neurophysiological assessment technology. In the applied sector, there will likely be an increased ability to identify valid neurophysiological indicators of performance to exploit affective, cognitive, and motivational states and evaluate the effectiveness of training techniques and the readiness of combat units. The hurdles that must be overcome in order to detect individual psychological states are high: They include a better understanding of neural plasticity and variability as well as real-time measurements of neural function with accurate spatial localization. Continued improvements in technology will facilitate the detection of psychological states. Although technology for assessing the effects of the peripheral nervous system on glandular function has been available for many years, technology for assessing the effects of the central nervous system has been developed more recently. For example, inexpensive, noninvasive endocrine assays and noninvasive high-density electroencephalography and functional brain imaging technology have progressed remarkably. Newer brain imaging technologies promising both high spatial and high temporal resolution of brain processes began to appear only in the past decade. It remains to be seen how technology will evolve and how it will aid in the detection of psychological states and lies by neurophysiological means.

Key Finding (Finding 2-2). The committee recognizes the IC's strong interest in improving its ability to detect deception. Consistent with the 2003 NRC study *The Polygraph and Lie Detection*, the committee uniformly agreed that, to date, insufficient, high-quality research has been conducted to provide empirical support for the use of any single neurophysiological technology, including functional neuroimaging, to detect deception.

Opinions differed within the committee concerning the near-term contribution of functional neuroimaging to the development of a system to detect deception in a practical or forensic sense. Committee members who conduct neuroimaging research largely agreed that studies published to date are promising and that further research is needed on the potential for neuroimaging to provide a more accurate method to determine deception. Importantly, human institutional review board standards require, at a minimum, that individuals not be put at any greater risk than they would be in their normal everyday lives. The committee believes that certain situations would allow such testing under "normal risk" situations; although the committee strongly endorses the necessity of realistic, but ethical, research in this area, it does not specify the nature of that research in this report.

Key Recommendation (Recommendation 2-1). The committee recommends further research on multimodal methodological approaches for detecting and measuring neurophysiological indicators of psychological states and intentions. This research should combine multiple measures and assessment technologies, such as imaging techniques and the recording of electrophysiological, biochemical, and pharmacological responses. Resources invested in further cognitive neuroscience research should support programs of research based on scientific principles and that avoid the inferential biases inherent in previous research in polygraphy.

Neuropsychopharmacology

Drugs available today can modulate and even control some aspects of human psychology. New types of psychopharmacological drugs and related delivery systems could increase the ability to harness a drug's effects to human psychology. Current models of brain and nervous system functioning can help to identify the likely psychological effects of known drugs. Changes in models of brain function may, however, create new and surprising ideas about how, when, where, or why drugs produce their effects; about what those effects are; about which chemicals are able to alter human functioning; and about ways to enhance, minimize, or counteract drug effects. It is important to realize that the drugs that changed psychiatry in the mid-twentieth century were not generally predicted by psychological or pharmacological models of their time. Rather, the history of neuropsychopharmacology illustrates how a particular cultural, medical, or research climate may fail to anticipate new drugs, new ways of using drugs, or new drug effects.

Neuropsychopharmacological research shows that drugs can be utilized to achieve or modulate abnormal, diseased, or disordered psychology and can also bring about normal, healthy, or optimal function. One new and important capability of neuropsychopharmacology is cognition enhancement. The United States and other countries are now devoting considerable research to the discovery and development of pharmacological cognition enhancers. Emergent technologies may allow new pathways for drug delivery in addition to new drugs or new uses for existing drugs. Nanotechnologies will allow delivery of drugs across the blood-brain barrier in ways not now possible. Finally, there is broad international interest in this kind of research; specifically, in Asia there is substantial research in drug delivery to the brain.

Research challenges include the identification of new targets for drugs, new methods of altering cell function, new drug delivery systems, strategies to direct or control drug effects, and attempts to achieve targeted psychological effects.

Key Finding (Finding 2-4). Technological advances will affect the types of neuropsychopharmacological drugs available and methods for drug delivery. For the IC, nanotechnologies that allow drugs to cross the blood-brain barrier, increase the precision of delivery, evade immune system defenses, evade metabolism, or prolong actions at cellular or downstream targets will be of particular importance. These technologies will increase the likelihood that various peptides, or other brain proteins, could ultimately be utilized as drugs. Development of antidotes or protective agents against various classes of drugs that could be used by an enemy force will also be important.

Functional Neuroimaging

Functional neuroimaging uses technology to visualize qualitative as well as measure quantitative aspects of brain function, often with the goal of understanding the relationships between activity in a particular portion of the brain and a specific task, stimulus, cognition, behavior, or neural process. Electroencephalography and magnetoencephalography measure localized electrical or magnetic fluctuations in neuronal activity. Positron emission tomography, functional magnetic resonance imaging, near-infrared spectroscopic imaging, and functional transcranial Doppler sonography can measure localized changes in cerebral blood flow related to neural activity. Positron emission tomography and magnetic resonance spectroscopy can measure regional modulation of brain metabolism and neurochemistry in response to neural activity or processes. These functional neuroimaging modalities are complementary and offer different windows into complex neural processes. Accordingly, simultaneous multimodal imaging is an emerging area of great interest for research, clinical, commercial, and defense applications.

Functional neuroimaging technologies are commonplace in research and clinical environments and are affecting defense policy. Their continued development and refinement are likely to lead to applications that go well beyond those envisioned by current cognitive neuroscience research and clinical medicine. Some very advanced work will occur outside the United States because some new technologies are first being deployed abroad. Advanced types of functional neuro-imaging technology are likely to be deployed in areas such as business, human performance, risk assessment, legal applications, intelligence, and the military.

Real-time, continuous readouts of neuroimaging results will become increasingly important for the IC and the Department of Defense (DOD), which will evaluate them for temporal sequences that indicate psychological or behavioral states. While predictions about future applications of technology are always speculative, emergent neurotechnology may well help to provide insight into intelligence from captured military combatants, enhance training techniques, enhance cognition and memory of enemy soldiers and intelligence operatives, screen terrorism suspects at checkpoints or ports of entry, and improve the effectiveness of human-machine interfaces in such applications as remotely piloted vehicles and prosthetics.

Key Finding (Finding 2-5). Functional neuroimaging is progressing rapidly and is likely to produce important findings over the next two decades. For the intelligence community and the Department of Defense, two areas in which such progress could be of great interest are enhancing cognition and facilitating training. Additional research is still needed on states of emotion; motivation; psychopathology; language; imaging processing for measuring workload performance; and the differences between Western and non-Western cultures.

Computational Biology Applied to Cognition, Functional Neuroimaging, Genomics, and Proteomics

Computing is used pervasively today in the fields of neuroscience and cognition for analysis and modeling. It is used to analyze the enormous amounts of data from genome sequencing, ribonucleic acid (RNA) expression arrays, proteomics, and neuroimaging and to correlate them with experimental results so as to eventually understand the biology of the nervous system and of cognition. In modeling, computing is used to express a hypothesis in concrete mathematical terms. The model is then simulated in an attempt to validate the hypothesis and/or make a prediction. Mathematical models of various dynamical qualities can be constructed and used to make predictions. Mathematical models have been used, for example, to correlate sleep and performance by measuring both and using the relationship to make a prediction. The distinction between modeling and analysis is not always clear because many types of data analysis make basic assumptions about the data fitting a specific model.

The larger issue is whether a cognitive system can be constructed in the next two decades that, while not precisely mimicking a human brain, could perform some similar tasks, especially in a particular environment. Success would be determined not by how closely the system resembled the brain in its mechanisms of action, but by the degree to which the system performed specific cognitive tasks the same way as a typical human operator. This search for what is known as artificial intelligence has for many decades been a goal of computing efforts.

Perhaps most revolutionary would be an intelligent machine that uses the Internet to train itself. Currently, the Internet is by far the closest we have come to a total database of knowledge. One can imagine an intelligent system that continuously monitors and processes not only accumulated knowledge but also public and nonpublic information on current events. Modern search engines do that in a way but serve more to catalog knowledge than to come to intelligent conclusions. However, if a system that reasoned like a human being could be achieved, there would be no limit to augmenting its capabilities. Many efforts, large and small, to reach this goal have not yet succeeded.

Key Finding (Finding 3-6). As high-performance computing becomes less expensive and more available, a country could become a world leader in cognitive neuroscience through sustained investment in the nurture of local talent and the construction of required infrastructure. Key to allowing breakthroughs will be the development of software-based models and algorithms, areas in which much of the world is now on par with or ahead of the United States. Given the proliferation of highly skilled software researchers around the world and the relatively low cost of establishing and sustaining the necessary organizational infrastructure in many other countries, the United States cannot expect to easily maintain its technical superiority.

Key Recommendation (Recommendation 3-1). The intelligence community, in collaboration with outside experts, should develop the capability to monitor international progress and investments in computational neuroscience. Particular attention should be given to countries where software research and development are relatively inexpensive and where there exists a sizeable workforce with the appropriate education and skills.

Distributed Human-Machine Systems

Advances in neurophysiological and cognitive science research have fueled a surge of research aimed at more effectively combining human and machine capabilities. Results of this research could give human performance an edge at both the individual and group levels. Though much of this research defies being assigned rigid boundaries between disciplines, for the sake of convenience the committee has organized its discussion into four areas:

• *Brain-machine interfaces.* This category includes direct brain-machine interfaces for control of hardware and software systems. Traditional human interface technologies, such as visualization (Thomas and Cook, 2005), are not considered in this report.
• *Robotic prostheses and orthotics.* Included here are replacement body parts (robotic prostheses) and mechanical enhancement devices (robotic orthotics) designed to improve or extend human performance in the physical domain.
• *Cognitive and sensory prostheses.* These technologies are designed to improve or extend human performance in the cognitive domain through sensory substitution and enhancement capabilities or by continually sensing operator state and providing transparent augmentation of operator capabilities.
• *Software and robotic assistants.* These technologies also are designed to improve or extend human performance in the physical and/or cognitive domains. However, unlike the first three areas, they achieve their effect by interacting with the operator(s) rather than as assistants or team members in the manner of a direct prosthetic or orthotic extension of the human body, brain, or senses. Agent-based technologies for social and psychological simulations are not considered in this report.

Research in artificial cognitive systems and distributed human-machine systems has been hampered by unrealistic programs driven by specific, short-term DOD and intelligence objectives. Another problem is the inadequacy of current approaches to research metrics. Resolving this problem would enable meaningful progress. Finally, the study of ethical issues related to the design and deployment of distributed human-machine systems is virtually in its infancy and this is deplorable given the great potential of such systems for doing good or harm.

Key Finding (Finding 3-7). Unlike in the domain of cognitive neurophysiological research, where the topics are constrained by certain aspects of human physiology and brain functioning, progress in the domain of artificial cognitive systems and distributed human-machine systems (DHMS) is limited only by the creative imagination. Accordingly, with sustained scientific leadership there is reason for optimism about the continued development of (1) specialized artificial cognitive systems that emulate specific aspects of human performance and (2) DHMS, whether through approaches that are faithful to cognitive neurophysiology, or through some mix of engineering and studies of human intelligence, or by combining the respective strengths of humans and automation working in concert. Researchers are addressing the limitations that made earlier systems brittle by exploring ways to combine human and machine capabilities to solve problems and by modeling coordination and teamwork as an essential aspect of system design.

Cultural Underpinnings of Neuroscience

Basic and applied social science research into various aspects of culture can help the IC to understand the current status of cognitive neuroscience research and anticipate the directions it might take over the next 20 years.[3] Using social and cultural modeling and frameworks to predict behavior and intentions in an intelligence and military context will require learning how cultural groups are organized. The IC's understanding of culture will be enhanced if it takes a pluralist and globalist view of how cultural groups are organized, and how research is conducted and applied in the field of culture studies. For example, research into intercultural management and leadership can warn IC and national security analysts not to assume that Western theories can be universally applied in multicultural situations. Concepts found in cultural research serve as intervening variables in neuroscience research, providing an understanding of how culture impacts human cognition and affect with respect to brain functioning, meaning, and behavior in diverse social and political situations.

Culturally accurate intelligence and strategic analysis have long been of interest to IC and national security analysts. Conventional social science models based primarily on Western ideas may be compromised by invisible biases. The need is growing to understand hearts and minds at a strategic level because of their potential to exacerbate insurgencies and other problems. Deficiencies in cultural knowledge at the operational level can also adversely affect public opinion. Likewise, ignorance of a culture at the tactical level could endanger both civilians and troops. Advances in inferring cross-cultural intention and meaning are possible with a comparative cultural research agenda. Cross-cultural comparative research can be pursued to test whether the brain function and human behavior assumed by European and U.S. psychological models are universal.

Key Finding (Finding 4-1). There is a growing awareness in the U.S. government that effective engagement in a complex world—commercially, militarily, and diplomatically—will increasingly require an unbiased understanding of foreign cultures. Research is enhancing understanding of how culture affects human

---

[3]For purposes of this report, "culture" is defined as a collective identity whose shared membership has distinct values, attitudes, and beliefs. Behavioral norms, practices, and rituals distinguish one cultural group from another. Distinct cultural groups are defined around regional, political, economic, ethnic, social, generational, or religious values.

cognition, including brain functioning, and is even suggesting a link between culture and brain development. The U.S. military is placing greater emphasis on cultural-awareness training and education as a critical element in its strategy for engaging in current and future conflicts. Military conflicts will increasingly involve prolonged interaction with civilian populations in which cultural awareness will be a matter of life and death and a major factor in outcomes. Similarly, political leaders, diplomats, intelligence officers, corporate executives, and academicians will need a deeper, more sophisticated understanding of foreign cultures to communicate more effectively with their counterparts in non-Western societies in the era of globalization.

Key Recommendation (Recommendation 4-1). The growing U.S. government interest in cultural training and education is well placed, and its investment in related research and development and in practical training should be substantially increased. Training programs, to be most effective, should be developed and implemented on a multidisciplinary basis. Investment should be made particularly in neuroscience research on the effects of culture on human cognition, with special attention to the relationship between culture and brain development.

Ethical Implications of Cognitive Neuroscience and Neurotechnology Evolution

Discussions of neuroethics and human experimentation for national security purposes generate unique concerns. The brain is viewed as the organ most associated with personal identity. There is sure to be enormous societal interest in any prospective manipulation of neural processes. Several internationally accepted documents guide the ethical treatment of human participants in biomedical research. The most authoritative is the World Medical Association's (WMA's) Declaration of Helsinki (DoH) (WMA, 1964). Although the international community largely accepts and respects the DoH, data on compliance by individual states are not available. The 1948 Universal Declaration of Human Rights in principle has global authority and is legally compelling, but is not invoked as frequently as the DoH in the context of human subject research despite its clear language about the ethical treatment of human subjects (United Nations, 1948). The oldest document, the 1947 Nuremberg Code,[4] is not often cited directly as a reference document but has served as the foundation for other guiding documents, including federal regulations in the United States. More recently, the Council for International Organizations of Medical Sciences issued the International Ethical Guidelines for Biomedical Research Involving Human Subjects (Council for International Organizations of Medical Sciences, 2002). While these guidelines

---

[4]*Trials of War Criminals before the Nuremberg Military Tribunals under Control Council Law No. 10*, Vol. 2, pp. 181-182. Washington, D.C.: U.S. Government Printing Office, 1949.

are very detailed, practical, and sensitive to cultural differences between nations, they do not have the same prominence as the DoH. Other documents, both national and international, offer more specific guidance on separate aspects of biomedical research (e.g., clinical trials, drug development).

The various guidelines reflect a consensus on some core beliefs, including that the research must be reviewed from an ethics standpoint before it is conducted; that the research must be justifiable and contribute to the well-being of society in general; that the risk-benefit ratios must be reasonable; that informed consent or voluntariness is needed; that there is a right to privacy; that accurate reporting of data is obligatory; and that inappropriate behaviors must be reported.

Individual nations may have their own, additional, ethical rules and regulations. The committee researched the existence and scope of such documents for two nations, Iran and China, and looked for evidence of research there into cognitive neuroscience and biotechnology, specifically for military uses. In Iran, detailed codes on medical ethics and biomedical research have been officially ratified, and international documents have also been formally endorsed. China states that it complies with the international instruments guiding research ethics. While there has been considerable talk in China about improved and more comprehensive guidelines for biomedical research with human subjects, no new documents have been ratified recently by the government.

Potential Intelligence and Military Applications of Cognitive Neuroscience and Related Technologies

Technology warning in the IC today is hampered by several factors, including the low priority it has among senior leaders; the paucity of resources invested by the community in internal science and technology capability; the continuing inadequate attention of management to the needs of IC analysts; and the need to establish close ongoing collaborations with analysts in other agencies, the scientific community at large, the corporate world, and academia, where the IC can find the most advanced understanding of scientific trends and their implications.

Although there are a handful of excellent joint research programs between the very best of U.S. universities and medical schools and foreign laboratories, programs that contain cognitive neuroscience research components or research programs are largely based on U.S. research and approaches. Relationships with foreign entities exist primarily to make use of low-cost infrastructure outside the United States, not to gain access to non-U.S. approaches and applications. These observations are not intended to impugn the IC's current programs for cognitive research; however, identifying foreign technology surprise in scientific areas that are not represented in U.S. research is, and will continue to be, extremely difficult.

Key Finding (Finding 5-1). International market forces and global public demand have created an impetus for neuropsychopharmacology and neurotechnology research that will lead to new technologies and drugs, particularly in areas of cognition and performance, that will include off-label uses. Off-label drug use can alert intelligence analysts to compounds, methods of administration, or risk factors that may be unknown in civilian or military medicine and can help identify profiles of unanticipated effects.

Key Finding (Finding 5-4). Rapid advances in cognitive neuroscience, as in science and technology in general, represent a major challenge to the IC. The IC does not have the internal capability to warn against scientific developments that could lead to major—even catastrophic—intelligence failures in the years ahead. An effective warning model must depend on continuous input from strong internal science and technology programs, strong interactive networks with outside scientific experts, and government decision makers who engage in the process and take it seriously as a driver of resources. All that remains a work in progress for the IC.

REFERENCES

Council for International Organizations of Medical Sciences. 2002. *International Ethical Guidelines for Biomedical Research Involving Human Subjects.* Geneva, Switzerland, November 2002. Available from http://www.cioms.ch/guidelines_nov_2002_blurb.htm. Last accessed June 8, 2008.

National Research Council (NRC). 2003. *The Polygraph and Lie Detection.* Washington, DC: The National Academies Press. Available from http://www.nap.edu/catalog.php?record_id=10420.

NRC. 2005. *Avoiding Surprise in an Era of Global Technology Advances.* Washington, DC: The National Academies Press. Available from http://www.nap.edu/catalog.php?record_id=11286.

Thomas, J.J., and K.A. Cook. 2005. Illuminating the path: The research and development agenda for visual analytics. Richland, WA: National Visualization and Analytics Center. Available from http://nvac.pnl.gov/agenda.stm#book. Last accessed January 10, 2008.

United Nations. 1948. Universal Declaration of Human Rights. Adopted and proclaimed by General Assembly Resolution 217 A (III) of 10 December 1948. Palais de Chaillot, Paris, December 1948. Available from http://www.un.org/Overview/rights.html.

World Medical Association. 1964. Declaration of Helsinki: Ethical Principles for Medical Research Involving Human Subjects. Adopted by the 18th World Medical Association General Assembly. Helsinki, Finland, June 1964. Available from http://www.wma.net/e/policy/b3.htm.

1

The Big Picture:
Bridging the Science and Technology
for the Decision Maker

INTRODUCTION AND STUDY ORIGIN

This is the third report in a series produced under the auspices of the National Research Council (NRC) Standing Committee on Technology Insight—Gauge, Evaluate, and Review (TIGER) and sponsored by the Defense Intelligence Agency's (DIA's) Defense Warning Office (DWO) (NRC, 2006, 2008). As did the two previous reports, the current report resulted from discussions between the TIGER standing committee and components of the U.S. intelligence community (IC). The overall series is intended to assist the IC in identifying global technology trends that may affect future U.S. warfighting capabilities.

An earlier report, *Avoiding Surprise in an Era of Global Technology Advances* (NRC, 2005), provided the IC with a methodology to gauge the potential implications of emerging technologies. The methodology has been widely accepted as a new tool for assessing potential future national security threats from these emerging technologies. As part of a continuing relationship with the TIGER standing committee, the IC identified neurophysiological research, and especially technologies associated with that research—the study and integration of cognitive neuroscience, psychology, sociology, and neuropsychopharmacology—as a field that could pose strategic implications for U.S. national security.[1] Box 1-1 provides the study statement of task.

---

[1] The label "cognitive" in the title and elsewhere in this report is used in the broad sense. Unless otherwise noted, it refers to the cognitive sciences in general and comprises psychological and physiological processes underlying human information processing, emotion, motivation, social influence, and development. It includes contributions from all directly related disciplines, including the behavioral and social sciences, neurogenetics, proteomics, philosophy, mathematics, computer science, and linguistics. The label "neuroscience" is also used in the broad sense (unless specified otherwise) to

---

Box 1-1
Statement of Task

In an effort to better understand, and therefore forecast, the international neuro-physiological and cognitive/neural science research landscape and its potential to affect U.S. future national security, an ad hoc NRC study committee will:

• Review the current state of today's work in neurophysiology and cognitive/neural science, select the manners in which this work could be of interest to national security professionals, and trends for future warfighting applications that may warrant continued analysis and tracking by the intelligence community,
• Use the technology warning methodology developed in the 2005 National Research Council report *Avoiding Surprise in an Era of Global Technology Advances* (NRC, 2005) to assess the health, rate of development, and degree of innovation in the neurophysiology and cognitive/neural science research areas of interest, and
• Amplify the technology warning methodology to illustrate the ways in which neurophysiological and cognitive/neural research conducted in selected countries may affect committee assessments.

Advances in neurophysiological research could lead to asymmetric advantages in detecting psychological states, including deception, and the pharmaceutical enhancement or degradation of individual and group performance, as well as the development of human-machine interfaces, any or all of which could give an individual a performance edge.

Military and intelligence planners are uncertain about the likely scale, scope, and timing of advances in neurophysiological research and technologies that might affect future U.S warfighting capabilities. For good or for ill, an ability to better understand the capabilities of the body and brain will require new research that could be exploited for gathering intelligence, military operations, information management, public safety, and forensics.

In developing a framework for assessing the applicable trends in physiological research, this study focuses on how such a framework might be used by IC analysts tasked to predict the behaviors of individuals and groups, including evaluation of the kinds of data available to them. The principal goal of the methodology used in this study was to permit IC analysts to objectively evaluate whether an institution, region, or country merits further investigation and, where possible, to specify the cognitive-behavioral and neuroscience discipline(s) involved. Committee members were selected who would be familiar in general terms with the global cognitive-behavioral research landscape and be knowledgeable about the

---

refer to processes that take place in systems such as the central nervous system (i.e., the brain and the spinal cord), and the somatic, autonomic, and neuroendocrine systems.

disciplines involved. Efforts were made to correlate deep scientific understanding of current and projected research results with the possibility of disruptive technologies arising from those results.

Worldwide interest in the cognitive-behavioral sciences (the study and integration of neuroscience, psychology, and sociology) is increasing as new technologies emerge. Some of the most exciting of these technologies access the brain using noncontact, noninvasive breakthroughs at the nexus of physics, imaging processing, and neurophysiology. However, claims reported in the media are often rife with hyperbole, ignoring well-known scientific caveats and including overstatements not based on peer-reviewed and replicated findings. While new technologies promise major social, communications, and, especially, medical breakthroughs, they are also pushing the envelope of ethics, privacy, and policy. Understandably, policy makers, military and intelligence professionals, and planners are confused about whether the advances will be as great as has been predicted.

To the extent that these advances can be realized, they will be used to improve the human condition. A better understanding of the capabilities of the brain will expose opportunities for applied research that could be exploited for legal and forensic, military and police/public safety, and information and intelligence purposes. Some research possibilities are being highlighted and may even be overtaking traditional academic research; others are being described in ways that may overstate their promise. Certain work, especially that being conducted in foreign laboratories, may parallel or even outstrip the traditional, peer-reviewed work being done in the West. This could lead to asymmetric advances outside traditional science, perhaps in the detection of deception, in the modification, enhancement, or degradation of individual and group performance, and in man–machine interfaces that amplify human capabilities.[2] Though the United States and Western Europe have historically led the world in cognitive neuroscience research, programs in other countries are clearly advancing rapidly as the result of increased international collaboration and financial support.

Many of these countries are believed to be directing their research resources toward certain niche areas, such as unconventional uses for pharmaceuticals; real-time brain-machine interfaces; far-field and noncontact brain imaging technologies; and fusion of advanced software and processing applied to nonmedical applications. The IC needs to survey the factors that will shape development of international cognitive-behavioral neuroscience research in all these contexts.

---

[2]The committee believes that traditional science is generally understood to consist of testing hypotheses in nature. One challenge the committee felt strongly about was the need for the military and the IC to comprehend hypothesis generation, at the same time understanding that not all countries approach science like the United States. Moreover, emergent research often turns out to be unpredictable—that is, unplanned discoveries reveal new hypotheses (hypothesis generation), which in turn provide new knowledge. In the future, the IC will need to watch nontraditional countries using nontraditional methods of discovery.

However, it needs to observe the resulting landscape from high up to obtain a clearer understanding of emergent technologies that might have unethical applications. The committee was primarily interested in identifying trends in today's cognitive-behavioral neuroscience research landscape that will anticipate the state of international research in the next two decades. This process of identification and extrapolation is grounded in the current state of the science in selected areas of cognitive neuroscience research. In developing the methodology, the committee considered the end user (analysts and predictors of the behaviors of individuals and groups), the data available to them, the desired output, and the unique aspects (if relevant) of neuroscience research. Intelligence analysts were available for consultation throughout the project in order to ensure that the methodology was realistically applied, given the limitations of the data sets.

WHAT DECISION MAKERS WANT TO KNOW

In the next two decades, the questions being asked by decision makers are likely to be similar to what they are now, although the answers may be different. The projection of power, deterrence, and achieving military objectives all have the same need for accurate information. One can imagine high-level Department of Defense (DOD) personnel asking the IC and the neuroscience community specific questions, the answers to which may have a variety of applications, such as the following:

• *Can cognitive states and intentions of persons of interest be read?* Decision makers might ask members of the IC a question such as this: "How can I know what someone knows?" In situations where it is important to win the hearts and minds of the local populace, it would be useful to know if they understand the information being given them. Do they believe it? As information is analyzed before making an important decision, particularly in situations that may call for risking American lives, IC neuroscientists will surely be asked how one can know if someone is telling the truth.

• *Can cognitive capacities be enhanced?* In the future, as soldiers prepare for conflict, DOD may call on the neurophysiology community to assist in maintaining the warfighting superiority of the United States. Commanders will ask how they can make their troops learn faster. How can they increase the speed with which their soldiers process large amounts of information quickly and accurately? How can the neurosciences help soldiers to make the correct decision in the difficult environment of wartime operations? Other abilities of a soldier that might need enhancement could include transferring information and ensuring its precision.

• *Can cognitive states and intentions be controlled?* Although conflict has many aspects, one that warfighters and policy makers often talk about is the motivation to fight, which undoubtedly has its origins in the brain and is reflected in peripheral neurophysiological processes. So, one question would be "How can we disrupt the enemy's motivation to fight? Other questions raised by controlling the mind: How can we make people trust us more? What if we could help the brain to remove fear or pain? Is there a way to make the enemy obey our commands?

- *Can cognitive states be used to drive devices?* This general question leads to specific questions about applications for limb and organ control, immobilization, and repair. Applications, both positive and negative, may also be imagined for interfering with the mind to enhance the senses of hearing, sight, smell, and touch. Alternatively, physical agents such as white noise could be used to impair one or more senses. In the area of neuropsychopharmacology, drugs could target specific sensory receptors, perhaps to enhance, perhaps to interfere.

REPORT STRUCTURE

This chapter provides an overview of cognitive-behavioral neuroscience research and poses a series of questions that decision makers will probably want answered. Chapter 2 provides detail on areas of interest selected by the committee. Chapter 3 builds on Chapter 2 by illustrating emerging areas of cognitive-behavioral neuroscience technologies. Chapter 4 showcases two disciplines, neuroethics and the cultural underpinnings of social neuroscience, that could assist intelligence analysts by providing a larger context beyond fixed definitions of cognitive-behavioral neuroscience. Chapter 5 includes committee assessments of various aspects of cognitive-behavioral neuroscience using the technology warning methodology described earlier in this chapter. Appendix C provides a full account and explanation of the methodology.

REFERENCES

NRC (National Research Council). 2005. *Avoiding Surprise in an Era of Global Technology Advances.* Washington, DC: The National Academies Press. Available from http://www.nap.edu/catalog. php?record_id=11286.

NRC. 2006. *Critical Technology Accessibility.* Washington, DC: The National Academies Press. Available from http://www.nap.edu/catalog.php?record_id=11658.

NRC. 2008. *Nanophotonics: Accessibility and Applicability.* Washington, DC: The National Academies Press. Available from http://www.nap.edu/catalog.php?record_id=11907.

2

Current Cognitive Neuroscience
Research and Technology:
Selected Areas of Interest

INTRODUCTION

Cognitive neuroscience and related technologies constitute a multifaceted discipline that is burgeoning on many fronts. Based on the expertise of its members, and realizing that it could not possibly cover the entire range of science within the discipline, the committee chose to discuss three specific areas of interest: (1) challenges to the detection of psychological states and intentions via neurophysiological activity, (2) neuropsychopharmacology, and (3) functional neuroimaging. Even then, the study's timeline made it impossible to provide an exhaustive review. Despite these limitations, however, the following discussions accurately depict the current state of cognitive neuroscience research in the selected fields. The chapter also serves as the scientific foundation for Chapter 3.

CHALLENGES TO THE DETECTION OF PSYCHOLOGICAL STATES AND INTENTIONS VIA NEUROPHYSIOLOGICAL ACTIVITY

Overview

There is little doubt that great progress has been made over the last quarter century, particularly the last 10 to 15 years, in understanding the physiological and neural bases for psychological processes and behavior. Furthermore, there is a high likelihood that more progress will be made as more sophisticated theoretical models are developed and tested using ever more sophisticated assessment technology. In the applied sector, scientists will probably be better able to identify valid neurophysiological indicators of performance. For example, modeling the human genome will help researchers to index affective, cognitive, and motivational states and evaluate the effectiveness of training techniques or to determine the readiness of combat units.

The vast majority of neuroscientific research has been conducted at the group, or aggregate, level rather than at the individual level, and this trend is likely to continue. To achieve sophisticated and highly sensitive neurophysiological assessment of psychological states at the individual level, many significant challenges must be overcome. At a minimum, the neurophysiological indicators will probably have to be individually "tuned" to each user, given the issues of individual variability and plasticity described below.

To accurately assess psychological states using neurophysiological measures, basic neurophysiological work needs to be accomplished over the next two decades. The committee identified and discussed a nonexhaustive list of issues that need to be addressed and questions that need to be answered. These included the nature of psychological states compared to "mind reading," the nature of neurophysiological and neural activity, and barriers to identification of mental states and intentions.

An important qualification about the parameters necessary for determining psychological state became apparent during the committee's deliberations—the end use of information about the inferred psychological state. Because technology to infer a psychological state or intention could be put to a broad range of alternative uses, it is important to recognize that acceptable levels of error depend on the differential consequences of a false positive or a missed identification. The technology being applied to determine psychological state could even be derived from an incomplete model of brain function as long as it had sufficient predictive power to accomplish the desired goal. For instance, one would not need a complete model of brain function to construct a brain–computer interface that could improve the self-piloting capabilities of unmanned air vehicles. But the tolerance for error will be much less if a technology is used to determine whether an individual is lying about an act of treason, because the consequences of an error will be greater.

The committee believes that it is critical to fully understand the relationship between neurophysiological markers and actual mental states when the application is the detection of deception.

Mind Reading and Psychological States

It has proven difficult since the beginning of modern psychology 150 years ago to achieve agreement, even among psychologists and other behavioral scientists, on explicit definitions of psychological constructs. Such agreement is important because most psychological constructs bear labels borrowed from common language. Dictionary meanings and usage tempt many scientists to assume that they know the scientific definition of a psychological construct without consulting the scientific literature, where such constructs are explicitly defined.

Typical didactic schemes for organizing psychological constructs imply a more rigid separation between them than actually exists and operates. Today, the main organizing constructs for understanding psychology at the individual level are *affect, cognition,* and *motivation.*[1] However, such organization does not necessarily reflect how affective, cognitive, and motivational processes interact. Indeed, attempting to understand each construct in isolation rather than the three as an interdependent triumvirate is to wander in an epiphenomenal domain rather than a realistic psychological domain. If scientists could, for example, accurately determine how a particular soldier processes information about a member of the enemy force (cognition), that knowledge would do very little to help us understand how the soldier will behave toward that enemy unless scientists also take into account how he or she feels about that enemy (affect) and how both constructs play into motivational processes.

When behavioral scientists ask *why* individuals behave in certain ways, they typically are asking a motivational question. During the first half of the twentieth century, psychologists focused on external environmental factors such as reinforcement to explain motivation. In the latter half of that century, they focused on internal processes to explain affect (moods and emotions) and cognition (information processing, memory) but without knowing details of the causal interconnections among the processes. Today, psychologists understand that behavior occurs between interrelated affective, cognitive, and motivational processes on the one hand and environmental factors and processes on the other. This complex set of interrelated factors must be understood and accounted for to detect a psychological state—that is, to "read" a mind—using any technology.

There has been growing use of the term "mind reading" in the popular press and in a few circumscribed areas of the Department of Defense (DOD). Because the precise meanings of the terms that are used to communicate understanding are critical to the scientific endeavor, the committee believes it is important that the DOD and IC communities understand what is meant in this study by "mind reading" and "psychological state." Mind reading typically refers to the capacity (imparted by an external mechanism—that is, some form of technology) to determine precisely what an individual is thinking or intending, whether or not the individual is willing to communicate that state of mind. As discussed below, to "read" minds scientists must understand how minds really work to come up with a technology that is of real use, and there are several formidable barriers to

---

[1]Individual psychology is also determined by important factors such as fundamental biological drives and programming of behavior, cognition, and affect by all levels of biology, including genes, proteins, receptors, synapses, and nuclei, among others. In addition, endogenous and genetic drivers dominate cognition, affect, and behavioral capability—for example, in human development, sleep and circadian rhythms of cognition and affect, eating, the need for social affiliation and for salt and water, sexual drive, aggression, and nurturing—and dominate human behavior. This section of the report discusses in some detail environmental factors relating to individual psychology, but this is not meant to de-emphasize the importance of biological factors such as the ones just described.

achieving such an understanding any time in the next two decades. In contrast, "psychological state" sometimes refers to a broad range of mental activities associated with cognition, affect, and motivation, but more often refers to a discrete and definable mental state, for example, sustained attention (cognition), anger (affect), or hunger (motivation). The committee believes that experimentation, with the careful control of any number of possibly confounding variables, will result in important progress toward understanding the nature of psychological states over the next two decades, using current and yet-to-be developed technologies. It must be understood, however, that much neuroscientific research still infers psychological state based on the experimental controls. Barriers to being able to read minds as well as the hurdles that must be overcome to accurately determine psychological state are discussed below.

The Nature of Neurophysiological Activity

The progress being made by scientific discovery in the field of biology is truly amazing, particularly at the molecular level. At the level of the neural system, however, current knowledge is more speculative. This is understandable given the complexity of the brain. Estimates are that each of the (approximately) 100 billion neurons in the brain synapses—that is, connects—with as many as 50,000 other neurons, making for a large and complicated control network that will likely take decades more of scientific work to map out.

This level of complexity also makes it unnecessary to identify neural centers of activity that are responsible for or associated with specific psychological "modules" of activity. It has been shown that although the neural activity in some brain loci appears to increase or decrease during specified mental activities, these brain loci represent only a small fraction of ongoing neural activity (Raichle, 2007). The rest of the brain is still active, and much more of the operation of the brain system must be understood to develop a firm scientific basis for reliably inferring psychological states.

Barriers to Identifying Psychological States and Intentions via Neural Activity

A science of the relations of mind and brain must show how the elementary ingredients of the former correspond to the elementary functions of the latter. (James, 1890)

The hurdles that must be surmounted in order to detect individual psychological states in a scientifically valid way are quite challenging. Here, several of these challenges are identified and discussed.

Technological Limitations and Advances

The impediment to detection of psychological states via neurophysiological states that is currently the most tractable is availability of technology to monitor and measure putative neurophysiological and neural processes with high spatial and temporal resolution. Although the assessment of peripheral somatic and autonomic systems has been possible for many years (Shapiro and Crider, 1969), advances in the assessment technology have come only recently. Inexpensive, noninvasive endocrine assays (Dickerson and Kemeny, 2004) and noninvasive, high-density electroencephalographic and functional brain imaging technology with high spatial and temporal resolution of brain processes have advanced rapidly. However, scientists must be cautious about what to expect of these technologies in the next quarter century. Technology is yielding new and powerful measurement tools. However, these tools will require sound scientific methods to be of benefit.

Errors in Logic and the Scientific Method

Given that the challenge set forth in the statement of task is to help the intelligence community (IC) and Department of Defense (DOD) "better understand, and therefore forecast, the international neurophysiological and cognitive/neural science research landscape," members of the committee believe that individuals who are not members of the neuroscientific community tend to make several common errors of logic when they interpret the findings of various technologies that are used to infer psychological states. These errors tend to occur because people misunderstand the relationship between the neurophysiological measurements and the actual mental state that the scientist is attempting to measure. A heightened awareness of the potential for such errors may help the IC and DOD make the best possible decisions when evaluating the scientific claims of researchers in other countries as well as the United States.

Furthermore, because technological innovation is as elemental to certain branches of neuroscientific investigation as the neuroscience itself is, the IC and DOD are likely to encounter two approaches to developing end-user applications of neuroscience, one favored mainly by neural and behavioral scientists, the other by engineers. Both approaches have their strengths, but when evaluating neuroscience, there are important differences. The first approach, as articulated by Cacioppo and Tassinary (1990a), places a premium on plausible scientific theory and the causal relationships underlying the psychological construct and the physiological index. This approach emphasizes the discovery of causal relationships so the theory can be refined and more and more precise hypotheses can be posited, helping to avoid misinterpretation of the data—that is, third-variable confounding, as discussed below. The second approach (the "engineering" one) is to propose, demonstrate, or purport that a given device or technology or method works from a signal detection point of view—for example, "with this technology we can tell when a pilot is too tired to fly with 92.3 percent accuracy." Any underlying causal model is secondary to the correlated effects. This approach is appealing, works well for many applications, and fits well with the DOD's proactive approach to problem solving. One significant problem with the largely atheoretical "engineering" approach in neuroscience is that it leaves one open to third-variable confounding, because without a model it is not possible to predict potential confounding. Furthermore, if problems do develop in implementation, there is no model from which to predict the next step. In contrast, the theory-based approach is one of successive approximations by which the underlying theory is continually refined and built upon through the use of models describing the underlying causal relationships.

Relationship Between Neurophysiological Measures and Psychological State

First and foremost, it is important that the reader understand the nature of neuroscientific investigation. When a neuroscientist is studying the biochemistry or the physics involved in brain function—changes in amino acids or the flow of ions, for example—these physiological changes are the phenomenon of interest and the focus of the study. However, when a neuroscientist is studying a psychological state such as attention or anger, changes in brain activity or chemistry are the *correlates*, or the means by which scientists study the mental state, which is the phenomenon of interest. Whereas physiological changes may regularly accompany a shift in mental state, scientists cannot assume that the mental state bears a one-to-one correspondence with the neural changes they are measuring. A discerning reader might argue, "But what if (and this is a very large *if*) scientists knew everything about how the brain functions, and knew how to measure it; would they then, in fact, be measuring mental states?" This line of reasoning, which is often followed by the lay community, is actually a philosophy of science known as reductionism. Reductionism, introduced by Descartes in the seventeenth century, argued that complex things can be fully explained and predicted by reducing them to the interactions of their parts, which are simpler or more fundamental things. He said that the world was a machinelike system that could be understood by taking apart its pieces, studying them, and then putting them back together to see the larger picture. Taken to its logical extreme, measuring the biological mechanisms associated with a mental activity would be equivalent to measuring the mental activity itself rather than just a correlate.

Although a reductionist philosophy of science is accepted in many areas of modern science, including much of physics, chemistry, and microbiology, reductionism to these levels of analysis has never taken hold in the behavioral sciences, probably with good reason. Although reductionists (see, for example, Wilson, 1998) believe that behavior can best be explained by genetic biology and/or the operation of neural control mechanisms, most other scientists argue that reductionist assumptions limit scientific understanding of complex systems.

If this is true, mental states may be more than the sum of their parts and may not be amenable to measurement even if the underlying neural activity is fully understood. Stated another way, mental states may emerge only at a psychological level of analysis and cannot be described in terms of purely neurophysiological activity even though the mental states are assumed to be caused by the brain. If reductionism is indeed correct, then at the current level of knowledge about the complexity of neural systems, science is indeed a very long way from being able to read minds from genetic or neural information.

This argument is important because neuroscientists realize that they are measuring the correlates of some mental state, not the mental state itself. As such, the issue of how closely the measures of neural activity map on to the mental state of interest (discussed below) becomes important. This point is of less concern to certain applications of technology to infer brain states (such as augmenting cognition to facilitate the piloting of unmanned aircraft), but it becomes critical when aspects of the psychological state can have legal ramifications, as, for example, in the determination of deception or intent to harm. The knowledge that scientists do not *know* that the neural activity corresponds one to one with the actual mental state (deceiving) must be weighed very carefully in these instances.

Mapping Measurements of Neurophysiological Activity to Psychological States

The most critical barrier to the identification of a psychological state from its neural signature is the fact that the neural activity underlying the psychological state subserves multiple tasks, so there can therefore be no one-to-one correspondence between neural activity and any psychological state. An excellent example of this point is that of deception detection, or credibility assessment. William Marston, the father of the polygraphy technique for deception detection, believed that there was a unique physiological response during deception. This has proved not to be the case, and few investigators since Marston, including current researchers investigating the use of neural activity measurements to infer deception, believed a unique signature associated with deception would ever be found. Whereas investigators expect to find some consistency in neural response during deception, they do not expect the activated neurons to fire only when the individual is being deceptive and at no other time. Rather, these same neurons are likely to also fire during other types of cognitive and emotional states besides deception (e.g., anxiety, dealing with a heavy cognitive load, inhibiting a pre-potent response). Whereas some low-level physiological processes may have a one-to-one correspondence with neural activation, no higher-order phenomenon on the order of a mental state has been found to have this type of neural pattern. Accordingly, researchers investigating the neural correlates of psychological states must control for many other variables, including other mental states, that could account for the neural activity they are measuring to be more certain that their results are indeed due to the construct under investigation (say, anxiety rather than deception or vice versa).

Fortunately, there is a very useful approach to proper inference between indexes and psychological constructs or states originally suggested by Cacioppo and Tassinary (1990b), who elucidated four types of neurophysiological index for psychological constructs: outcomes, concomitants, markers, and invariants. Awareness of this typology helps us to recognize important inferential problems associated with putative neurophysiological and neural indices of psychological states. Whereas the goal of a neurophysiological index for a psychological construct may be a symmetric, one-to-one relationship between the index and the variable based on a plausible and verifiable scientific theory, in practice this is rare.[2] To be symmetric, the presence of the variable must always be accompanied by the presence of the index and vice versa, and the two must covary systematically. To be based on a plausible scientific theory, the underlying causal relationships between the psychological construct and the physiological index should be valid ones.

More commonly, neurophysiological indices are outcomes and concomitants. Outcomes and concomitants are merely associations or correlations between a physiological response (or set of responses) and a psychological construct that are context bound or context free, respectively (see Figure 2-1).

Neither enjoys a symmetric one-to-one relationship between the response and the construct. For instance, the sympathetically driven autonomic responses indicative of stress is an outcome within the Cacioppo and Tassinary framework (1990b)—that is, it is context dependent and asymmetric. In a different context (the diagnostic one Erasistratus found himself in), such responses could be related to different psychological states (e.g., love or anxiety).

Markers and invariants are associations between a physiological response and a psychological construct that are context-bound or context-free, respectively, but do enjoy a symmetric one-to-one relationship (Figure 2-1). There are few (see below) well-validated symmetric peripheral or central nervous system (CNS) neurophysiological markers of affective, cognitive, and motivational psychological constructs. This paucity is partially due to poor/insufficient understanding of how neurophysiological systems operate and the resulting lack of sophisticated and validated biopsychosocial theory, which have facilitated the development of valid markers and invariants of psychological states.

Symmetric (one-to-one correspondence) relationships have rarely, if ever, been shown to exist between psychological constructs and their neurophysiological indicators. This lack of a symmetric relationship is a major problem for

---

[2]"Symmetric" means "If A then B *and* if B then A." For example, if there is a symmetric relationship between a lie (A) and a neurophysiological response (B) then every time the lie occurs the specific neurophysiological response occurs *and* every time the neurophysiological response occurs the lie occurs. "Asymmetric" means "If A, then B, but not vice versa." For example, if a lie is accompanied by a neurophysiological response that does not mean every time the neurophysiological response occurs that a lie has occurred.

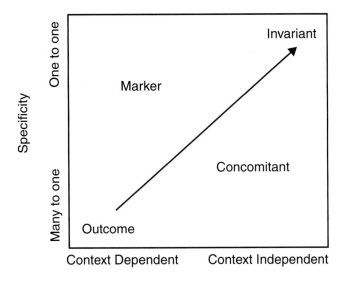

FIGURE 2-1 Associations between a physiological response (or set of responses) and a psychological construct. SOURCE: Cacioppo and Tassinary (1990b) ©1990 by the American Psychological Association. Adapted with permission. The use of APA information does not imply endorsement by the APA.

detecting psychological states from the indicators. Neurophysiological and neural activities are almost always multifunctional when it comes to causing underlying psychological constructs. So, even if every time an individual enters a psychological state (e.g., "love") the same portion of cortex (i.e., the left prefrontal cortex) is activated, does not mean that every time that portion of the cortex is activated the person is in that psychological state—that is to say, neurological measures may be sensitive, but are rarely specific. Good science avoids this logical error known as the "affirmation of the consequent."

These errors of inference can be avoided by precisely specifying the circumstances or "controls" under which the data can be interpreted by limiting the number psychological states. For instance, a brain–computer interface designed to assess attention to an external task and that has been accompanied by individual training for the user may place sufficient limits on both the environment and the user's possible states to allow accurate and useful interpretation of the neural responses. This highly controlled scenario, however, which has controls similar to the experimental controls that are used to interpret neuroimaging data does not amount to mind reading or to determining intent from the raw neural signals. Rather, a cognitive state is inferred based on the controls placed on the situation and is still subject to potential signal detection errors (e.g., false positives, false negatives, misses).

Avoiding Errors of Inference

Fortunately, a reductionist philosophy of science is not a requisite for drawing valid inferences about psychological states from neurophysiological and neural activity if one accepts the "identity thesis" as a basic metaphysical assumption. This assumption states that all psychological phenomena occur via bodily processes and is widely shared by behavioral scientists and neuroscientists (Cacioppo and Tassinary, 1990a; Blascovich, 2000; Blascovich and Seery, 2007). Accordingly, there is nothing ethereal about human behavior, and all psychological states are embodied somehow. If one can associate certain neurophysiological data with certain psychological states, then identifying psychological states from such information is a potentially tractable, though very difficult, challenge. Several logical and inferential issues, including those associated with the section below on the third variable problem, cause this challenge to be daunting.

The Third Variable Problem. When two variables, such as a psychological state and some specified neurophysiological measure, are related probabilistically, even if perfectly so, scientists cannot assume that they are causally related. For example, the correlation between shoe size and reading ability in children might be a spurious correlation. There is no doubt that both increase with age; however, correlation does not imply causality. Correlation is necessary for causality, but two other criteria must be met to imply causality: (1) time ordering (the cause must occur before the effect) and (2) third variables must be ruled out. Whereas an engineering approach can be used to determine time sequencing, a scientific model could allow ruling out third variables as the cause of a correlation; however, a poor or incomplete model will allow for many interpretations of an effect that might have an altogether different cause. This becomes a significant problem, for instance, when one wishes to decide whether a person is lying on a polygraph test; even if there is a high correlation between guilt and strong autonomic reactions to certain questions, it would be a mistake to conclude that guilt is causing the stronger reactions if anxiety, not guilt, can produce those same reactions.

The goal of a neurophysiological index of a psychological construct is a symmetric, one-to-one relationship between the index and the variable based on a plausible and verifiable scientific theory. To be symmetric, the variable must always be accompanied by the index and vice versa, and the two must covary systematically. To be based on a plausible scientific theory, the underlying causal relationships between the psychological construct and the physiological index should be valid.

Brain Plasticity

Brain plasticity refers to changes that occur in brain organization and function as a result of experience. There is now considerable evidence that brain activity associated with a psychological state or process can change throughout life as a function of factors such as sleep, maturation, experience, damage, exogenous (e.g., pharmacological) agents or a combination of these. Indeed, most poststroke rehabilitation therapy (e.g., relearning walking, talking) would be ineffective if such change were not possible.

Brain plasticity is manifested in at least three ways. One involves functional shifts and changes that occur when control of motoric behavior reorganizes itself in a different area of the cortex as a result of experience. A second way, termed synaptic plasticity, involves changes in neuroreceptor production and/or sensitivity that potentiate or antagonize the likelihood of synaptic transmission. A third way, at least speculatively, brain plasticity may manifest itself is changes in brain structure; that is, actual changes in the number of neurons and synapses, the most obvious examples of which are increases occurring early in life and decreases occurring as a result of lesions or aging.

Brain plasticity represents a challenge to those seeking to develop neuronal indexes for psychological states—i.e., outcomes, concomitants, markers, and invariants—on an individual level, because structural, organizational, and functional differences between individuals—and within them over time—will have to be accounted for. It is also possible that a high degree of plasticity-based error in any given index could reduce its sensitivity and specificity and, hence, its practical value for "reading" individual minds. However, this remains an open question, for scientists do not yet know how plasticity might affect any given set of measures across various populations.

Variability Within and Between Individuals

Two important challenges to using brain states to index psychological states are variability between individuals and also within a single individual. It seems likely that brain plasticity, along with genomic factors, may be one of the underlying causes of such variability, which apparently exists. However, "it is not easy to change the habits of people who are comfortable with traditional ways of doing things, and developers of cognitive models have continued to rely for support mainly on the fitting of functions such as curves of learning, retention, and generalization to averaged data" (Estes, 2002).

Estes has examined the relationships between typical brain scan images aggregated across individuals and those of the individual cases from which aggregated images are derived. Figure 2-2 illustrates the problem of individual variability for location of episodic memory in the brain. The leftmost image is the group or aggregate image. The next three images illustrate some of the individual cases from which the aggregate image was derived. None of the individual images match the group image. Hence, it would be inappropriate to base a neural index of the operation of episodic memory on the aggregate picture without adjustment for individual differences.

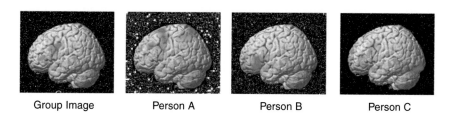

Group Image   Person A   Person B   Person C

FIGURE 2-2 Individual variability in the case of the putative location of episodic memory in the brain. SOURCE: Reprinted with permission from unpublished work (Miller, 2007).

Miller concludes that "investigations into the sources of unique individual brain activity may be necessary in order to understand the dynamic patterns of brain activity that underlie widely distributed, strategy-filled tasks like episodic memory" (Miller, 2007). There appears, moreover, to be variability across tasks, with some tasks showing more or less variability of locus than others. Furthermore, Miller reported that within-subject location appeared to be relatively stable across time, such that the same areas were activated in the same individual by the same task performed 6 months apart (Miller et al., 2002a,b). Individualized approaches to functional mapping, however, are feasible under certain circumstances. For instance, if a government wanted to outfit trained combat pilots flying high-tech aircraft with some type of neural interface, it would make sense to invest in determining individualized neurophysiological markers. Accounting for individual variability is both reasonable and feasible, because within-subject variability across time (after accounting for reorganization due to learning) tends to be low for cognitive tasks (Miller, 2007). This cost-benefit argument is more of a problem when attempting to apply a generic (averaged) algorithm to a given individual without individual tuning.

Specificity of Psychological States Within Contexts

The likelihood of developing valid neurophysiological indexes for inferring psychological states or intentions depends on the required specificity of the state itself and the specificity of the context within which it occurs. It is typically easier to develop an accurate index of a given psychological state if the number of candidate states can be limited by experimental controls. Consider, as an example, a vigilance scenario in the cognitive domain. It would be simpler to develop a neurophysiological index that marks a person as consciously processing information at a general level (e.g., having or not having the resources to cope with the situation he or she is in) than at a more specific level (e.g., having or not having specific resources). In the affective domain, it would be simpler to develop an index that distinguishes the polarity of a superordinate affective state (e.g., negative versus positive) than an index that distinguishes between more specific superordinate states (e.g., anger or fear). In the motivational domain, it would be easier to develop an index that distinguishes between fairly general superordinate motivational states (e.g., avoidance or approach) than to develop one that distinguishes more specific states (e.g., take flight or surrender).

Simultaneously indexing superordinate categories of general cognitive, affective, and motivational psychological states based on neurophysiological information can have great practical value because these general categories of psychological states are highly interdependent and simultaneous. Hence, if one could index all three categories simultaneously in a given context (say, warfighting), the resulting combined index would be more useful for drawing inferences and making predictions than any single index. Furthermore, one would be able to make these predictions without asking the warfighter questions and one could refine the predictions to reflect these continuously available indexes.

Indeed, one can probably infer psychological or behavioral intentions more accurately based on the combination index. If the cognitive index revealed that a soldier evaluates his or her resources as sufficient to meet the perceived needs in the particular context (e.g., a battle), if the affective index revealed that the soldier is experiencing positive affect (e.g., challenge) rather than negative affect (e.g., threat), and if the motivational index revealed that the soldier is motivated to approach rather than avoid the situation, one would could reasonably conclude that the soldier was prepared or even intended to do battle. On the other hand, if one index revealed that the soldier cognitively evaluates his or her resources as insufficient, another revealed that he or she is experiencing negative affect, and a third revealed that the soldier is avoidance-oriented, one could reasonably conclude that the individual was ready to retreat.

Existing peripheral neurophysiological measures include the following: (1) hemodynamic markers of cognitive resource/demand evaluations—for example, reciprocal changes in cardiac output and total peripheral resistance (Blascovich and Tomaka, 1996), (2) electromyographic indexes of affect—for example, relative reciprocal increases and decreases in zygomaticus major and corrugator supercillii muscle movements in the face (Cacioppo et al., 1986), and (3) cardiac indexes of approach/avoidance motivation—for example, increases or decreases in cardiac ventricular contractility and heart rate (Blascovich and Tomaka, 1996). If one could develop CNS indexes of superordinate categories of cognitive, affective, and motivational state, there would be a useful redundancy.

Assumptions About Base Rates of Psychological States and Intentions

Just as they like to rely on averaged data (Estes identified this propensity in 2002), many scientists also assume that base rates of dichotomous psychological states are 50/50. Much as scientists know that not everyone or every brain is average, they also realize that the probability that a person will act in one way rather than another is not necessarily 50 percent. This realization notwithstanding, development and even validational work on indexes of psychological states often assumes a base rate of 50 percent.[3]

If base rates of psychological states, such as intentions to commit an act of terrorism or to defect, were 50 percent, individuals with such intentions would be much easier to identify. Unfortunately, many important psychological states are infrequent events, with the consequence that indexes validated assuming a 50 percent base rate produce a very large number of mistaken detections. Green and Swets's classic paper on signal detection theory (1966) detailed the logic and mathematics for inferring the existence of target states from signals (or indexes) as a function of base rates.

Mistaken detections can be avoided only when a target signal is in almost perfectly symmetric (i.e., 1 to 1) correspondence with the target event in the biological or other system. Additionally, systems for transmitting and identifying the target signal must be almost perfectly accurate (Imrey, 2007). Imrey further argues that (1) combinations of these two circumstances are rare; (2) intuition on this point is notoriously poor, partly because of the ways accuracy is commonly expressed; (3) known biases in data collection invariably lead to overoptimism; (4) overoptimism means overconfidence in the reliability of results, and (5) this means underestimation of false positives and false negatives. A specific discussion on base rates and the detection of deception is found later in the chapter under the case study of detecting deception.

Finding 2-1. Cognitive neuroscientists can identify neurophysiological markers of general psychological states—for example, positive versus negative affect, automatic versus controlled cognitive processing, approach versus avoidance motivation, attention versus inattention—within individuals in specified contexts but are not yet able to identify highly specific psychological states and intentions—that is, exactly what a particular person is thinking, intending, or doing. Given the current state of knowledge about brain neurophysiology, it is highly likely that any advances in collective knowledge about individual psychological states over the next two decades will continue to occur in highly controlled situations where the number of candidate mental states is limited. The ability to determine a person's mental state strictly from neurophysiological markers without environmental controls is unlikely to be gained any time in the next two decades.

---

[3]In the experimental literature, and especially in the lie detection literature, tacit assumption of 50 percent appears to guide much of the physiological indexing of psychological states. The committee notes this rate may seem otherwise high.

Detection of Deception as an Example of Efforts to Identify Accurate Neurophysiological Indexes of Specific Psychological States in Individuals

The concept of the detection of deception was recently broadened and is now known as "credibility assessment," and includes additional factors such as source verification and witness corroboration. The concept is of considerable interest to the IC and DOD. Detection of deception can serve to illustrate the considerations discussed above as barriers to the identification of accurate neurophysiological indices of specific psychological states in individuals (Feinberg and Stern, 2005).

At the societal level, the capacity to detect deception is valued for many social, legal, and medical reasons. At the government level, the capacity to detect deception is valued because those having or seeking authority and/or power need to be able to safeguard the national interest. At the individual level, detection of deception helps to identify individuals who threaten some important value of a social group. In addition, it often makes sense to help determine the reliability of information or witnesses before resources are allocated. As such, technologies for the detection of deception entail identifying a specific kind of psychological state at the individual, or idiographic, level.

Not unlike in the scientific community at large, there was considerable debate among members of the committee about the ability to develop useful neurophysiological markers of deception. The committee believed, however, that it is critical for the IC and DOD to understand where opinions differed. Box 2-1 summarizes the key points of agreement and disagreement on detection of deception.

Previous Research on Detection of Deception

No known lie-detection technology has been sufficiently accurate (i.e., virtually inerrant) to be legally acceptable, especially given the relatively low base rates for many types of threats to a social order. As described above, the main technology used during the last 100 years in the United States and a few other countries (e.g., Israel, Canada, and Japan) is the polygraph, the generic name for an instrument that can record multiple physiological measurements which has come to be closely associated with the lie detection technique utilizing it. Conventional polygraphy relies on psychophysiological measures of the sympathetic nervous system response (respiration rate, heart rate, electrodermal activity) to detect anxiety associated with guilt or lying (OTA, 1990). As determinants of psychological states, however, these autonomic response suffer, in particular, from a lack of specificity and cannot differentiate guilt from other cognitive/affective states—say anxiety—resulting in an unacceptably high level of false positives (Office of Technology Assessment, 1983; Iacono, 2000). A report on the polygraph and lie detection (NRC, 2003, p. 4) concluded that:

. . . in populations of examinees such as those represented in the polygraph research literature, untrained in countermeasures, specific-incident [i.e., criminal] polygraph tests can discriminate lying from truth telling at rates well above chance but below perfection.

However, this should not be understood to be the applied accuracy of polygraph testing in operational field situations. Readers should note that many of the examinees referred to in the quote above are research subjects who, for the most part, are often informed of the nature of the research beforehand and are not typically drawn from the population to whom polygraph tests are typically given (individuals being investigated for criminal activity, those seeking employment in sensitive national security positions, prisoners of war). Often participants are college students or other volunteers and are hardly representative of populations that are likely to threaten the social order. Hence, the NRC report goes on to conclude that "polygraph testing yields an unacceptable choice for . . . employee security screening between too many . . . employees falsely judged as deceptive and too many major security threats left undetected" (NRC, 2003, p. 6).

It is the lack of specificity, in particular, of these autonomic measures to discriminate deception from other affective states that leads to insufficient positive and negative predictive power. That is, autonomic responses, at least as measured by the polygraph, are "outcomes" only, could represent a number of psychological states, and must be interpreted within a highly specified context. It is not surprising, then, that both the IC and the DOD have been interested in more precise (more sensitive and specific) measures of deception detection. As for other deception detection techniques, the report concluded that:

Some potential alternatives to the polygraph show promise, but none has *yet* been shown to outperform even the polygraph. None shows any promise of supplanting the polygraph for screening purposes in the near term. (NRC, 2003, pp. 7-8)

However, the report (NRC, 2003, p. 174) goes on to state that:

Functional brain imaging techniques have important advantages over the polygraph, in theory, because they examine directly what the brain is doing. . . . Not enough is yet known about the specific cognitive or emotional processes that accompany deception, about their localization in the brain, or about whether imaging signals can differentiate the brain activity associated with these processes from brain activity associated with other processes to make an assessment of the potential validity of these techniques on the grounds of the basic science. Further research with fMRI, coupled with a scientifically based cognitive psychological approach to deception, will be needed to determine if these issues can be addressed. . . . If a research effort is undertaken to find improved scientific techniques for the detection of deception, basic research on brain imaging would be a top candidate for the research agenda.

Box 2-1
Committee Agreements and Disagreements on
Detection of Deception

Agreement

The committee agreed that, as outlined in previous NRC reports, traditional measures of deception detection technology have proven to be insufficiently accurate. Second, the committee agreed that the IC and DOD should understand the nature of the relationship between neural/physiological/cognitive measures of brain states and the psychological states they are meant to measure. This derived from the concern that the neural correlates of deception could be construed as incontrovertible evidence of deception and therefore (mistakenly) used as the sole evidence for making critical legal decisions with lasting consequences. Current physiological measurements cannot be taken as direct measures of psychological states. Third, the committee agreed that for large-scale screening, the low-base-rate problem—very few terrorists among millions of travelers—created a significant problem given current rates of reliability. Fourth, the committee agreed that even if a highly reliable deception test were developed, it should be treated as only one element in a Bayesian approach. Fifth, the committee agreed that future research on measures of deception would benefit from a scientific, theory-driven approach in concert with an applied, problem-oriented approach. Lastly, the committee agreed that insufficient high-quality research using an appropriate research model and controls has been conducted on new modalities of credibility assessment to make a firm, data-driven decision on their accuracy.

Disagreement

The committee disagreed on whether functional brain measurements would prove to be more reliable for detecting deception than traditional autonomic polygraphy. Detractors cited neural plasticity, individual variability, and low base rates as barriers to developing accurate indices of deception. In contrast, several committee members who conduct functional magnetic resonance imaging (fMRI) and functional near-infrared spectroscopy (fNIRS) imaging research agreed that preliminary studies of deception using these modalities were promising because they found consistent results across research protocols, technologies, and populations. Second, the committee disagreed on what level of accuracy would be a useful or practical for detecting deception. Some committee members believed that because of the base-rate problem and the legal implications of deception, accuracy rates should be virtually inerrant to be practical, whereas others believed that measurements that kept the error rate to 1 percent or less would be useful if combined with the Bayesian approach. Lastly, the committee disagreed on whether more financial resources should be put into further research on deception detection. Some members strongly believed more research resources were warranted, others strongly disagreed.

For illustrative purposes, the committee next discusses deception detection work in light of the challenges described above. As noted, there was considerable debate among the committee members about what would constitute a practical or useful application of technology to the assessment of psychological states.

Deception and the Nature of Neurophysiological Measures

Understanding the nature of the relationship between physiological markers and the psychological states that are purportedly assessed by quantifying the markers is critical for several reasons. First, users of the technology must recognize the limitations of the tools they are using. The majority of polygraphers do not make the mistake of believing that they are measuring deception directly via neurophysiological information, avoiding an unwarranted reductionistic approach. Rather, they claim that certain neurophysiological changes (e.g., respiration, heart rate, blood pressure, electrodermal activity), as a set, pattern themselves differently during acts of deception than during acts of truth telling. This places a burden on the methods used to gather the psychophysiological or neurological data, as proper interpretation of the data fundamentally relies on appropriate methodological technique and controls.

While it can be tempting to assume that brain imaging or other neurophysiological measurements allow direct access to the psychological state under investigation, this assumption is not warranted. Based on research to date, it is highly improbable that there is any specific "lie circuit" in the brain that is dedicated to deception. Rather, the neural circuits that respond during deception will respond in other, nondeceptive circumstances, and only appropriate techniques will allow accurate interpretation of the data. The committee agrees that important legal decisions should not be made as if incontrovertible proof of deception existed if they are based only on the correlates of deception.

Unfortunately, the biopsychosocial theory underlying the putative relationships between the autonomic measures that are obtained with a traditional polygraph and their actual value as accurate indices of lying remains unsophisticated and essentially unchanged for nearly a century. Twenty-five years ago (1983), the United States Office of Technology Assessment issued a report prepared by a group of scientists who had evaluated the scientific validity of polygraph testing for lie detection (OTA, 1983). The report concluded that "the basic theory of polygraph testing is only partially developed and researched. . . . A stronger theoretical base is needed for the entire range of polygraph applications" (NRC, 2003, p. 6).

This statement largely reflects the paucity of well-designed and controlled studies for investigating the potential confounds when a strong inference is drawn from polygraphy data collected under a great variety of conditions. From a neuroscientific perspective, theory must be refined through experimentation. The report leveled the same criticism at the theoretical basis of polygraphic lie detection (NRC, 2003). Indeed, a long line of similar reports, including one in the archives of the National Research Council as early as 1917 and another in 1954 (Guertin and Wilhelm, 1954), made the same point.

This may be due to the fact that there are essentially two communities when it comes to judging the utility of the polygraph in determining deception, the polygraph community and the scientific community (Porges, 2006). These two communities base their judgments on different criteria. A critical difference between them has been their approach to research: The polygraph community has long taken an applied, problem-oriented approach, with efficacy as its goal, driven by perceived societal needs. The scientific community, in contrast, takes a basic, theory-driven approach that emphasizes understanding the mechanisms underlying the process of deception, driven by the principles of science as they relate to society. These two approaches are often conceptualized as inherently divergent, which they certainly have been in practice. However, lacking a scientific basis, the applied approach has failed to increase its efficacy or advance its credibility over several decades, as outlined above.

The literature on lie-detection research, which has long focused mostly on measurements of autonomic reactions, appears to value seemingly high correlations between particular neurophysiological responses and the prevarication they identify, independent of sound biopsychosocial theory. Continued reliance on a century-old, outdated physiology-based rationale has resulted in a failure to advance the underlying science. The best that can be said for the current physiological indexes of lying used in polygraph testing is that they are outcomes, the type of index that provides the logically weakest basis for inference (Cacioppo and Tassinary, 1990b). Put even more succinctly, the lack of biopsychosocial theoretical sophistication underlying polygraphic lie detection techniques over the past century has led to entropy in the field of lie detection. Because no known physiological or neurophysiological measure enjoys a one-to-one relationship with deception, all correlates of deception have multiple causes, only one of which is deception. This being the case, protocols and uses that rely on very few or even a single response to determine deception will be highly susceptible to false positives, despite which such protocols continue to be used (see, for example, Tsiamyrtzis et al., 2007). This has been demonstrated many times from work in such fields as event-related potentials, where multiple trials have proved much more reliable than single trials. If a marker is a true correlate of the deceptive state, it should survive several response trials, capitalizing on Bayesian probability. (Although it is well known that autonomic responses habituate, they can serve as markers for a few trials.)

The committee agrees that an integration of basic, theory-driven science with an applied, problem-oriented approach could facilitate acceptable solutions to the assessment of credibility. According to Porges (2006), basic science can help delineate the neural processes underlying deception and the theoretical relationships among the psychological state(s), their neural and physiological markers, their measurement, and their application in the field.

Improvements in Technology

Given that standard polygraph technology is no different in basic measurement principles than it was a century ago and, according to the literature, has failed to produce sufficient reliability, it is not surprising that many lie-detection researchers have turned to newer CNS assessment technologies, including high-density electroencephalography, near-infrared spectroscopy (fNIRS), and functional magnetic resonance imaging (fMRI) to improve the accruracy with which it detects lies. A small formative body of published research on the neural circuitry associated with deception utilizes various neuroimaging techniques. Recent studies using positron emission tomography (PET) and fMRI have provided insights into the neural circuitry associated with deception, with specific areas in the prefrontal cortices and amygdala being the most commonly implicated regions (Abe et al., 2006, 2007; Mohamed et al., 2006; Davatzikos et al., 2005; Langleben et al., 2002, 2005; Lee et al., 2002, 2005; Nuñez et al., 2005; Phan et al., 2005a; Kozel et al., 2004a,b, 2005; Ganis et al., 2003; Spence et al., 2001). Recent fNIRS studies of deception have also implicated prefrontal brain regions in the neural circuitry associated with deception (Bunce et al., 2005). Consistent with the Bunce et al. (2005) observation, through the end of 2007, all published neuroimaging studies of deception except one (Langleben et al., 2002), including PET, fNIRS and fMRI technologies, studies of well-practiced vs. spontaneous lies (Ganis et al., 2003), studies of malingering, and cultural samples (Lee et al., 2005, with Chinese subjects, Bunce et al., 2005, with East Indian subjects) have found activation in a similar area of the dorsolateral/ventrolateral prefrontal cortex. Another recently published study correlated fMRI images with standard skin conductance measurements during a concealed information paradigm, with interesting results (Gamer et al., 2007). Although some members of the committee believed this preliminary body of work to be quite promising there has not yet been sufficient systematic research to determine if functional neuroimaging can meet the challenges to the neurophysiological detection of psychological states relevant to deception, as described above. Future research is warranted in the brain plasticity and variability; specificity of psychological states; and base rates.

Brain Plasticity and Individual Variability

An important divergence between traditional polygraphic lie detection and newer lie detection based on newer CNS assessment technologies is the latter's susceptibility to problems created by the brain's plasticity and resultant individual variability in CNS structure and function. For example, if the loci of CNS synaptic transmissions underlying prevarication vary across individuals or within an individual across time, those loci would not be accurate enough to be useful as neurophysiological indexes of lying for individual testing. This is still an open question because to date, no sufficient research on these issues has been published. If individual variability proves to be a significant factor, there will be no scientific basis for using the newer assessment technologies unless theoretical mechanisms relating such variability to the biopsychsocial basis for lying can be specified and validated. This does not mean that a theory could not be developed, and some preliminary models have already been proposed (Porges, 2006; Spence, 2004). However, a great deal of appropriate research needs to be done before a specific conclusion could be drawn about the validity of CNS measures of intentional deception, with an interactive process between the scientific model and the research. While this does not rule out any role for an applied, problem-oriented approach—for example, does the outcome or marker predict at a given level of sensitivity/specificity—a good model would help to avoid serious misinterpretation of the data.

In addition to CNS-based measurement, several other sensing techniques are being investigated for their potential ability to discern deception or concealed knowledge. These techniques may avoid some of the issues surrounding neural plasticity, but they must still meet appropriate criteria for accuracy. Some are remote, noncontact sensing techniques that measure autonomic function and are already in use. For instance, laser Doppler vibrometry is a remote sensing technique for heart rate, blood pressure, and several other physical properties. Although the technique does provide more information about heart function than a polygraph, it typically measures aspects of autonomic function associated with stress in response to threat. Other similar techniques include voice stress analysis, pupilometry, and infrared measures of the periorbital regions.

One measurement that appears to have a largely cognition-based etiology is that of eye-movement-based memory assessment (EMMA) (see, for example Marchak, 2006). This method is based on evidence that people scan faces they have previously seen in a different way than they scan novel faces (Altoff and Cohen, 1999). People reliably use fewer eye fixations, sample fewer regions, and fewer statistical constraints in viewing familiar rather than new faces. By tracking and quantifying these eye movement patterns using the appropriate technology and experimental controls, researchers can identify concealed knowledge. These patterns can also be combined with performance measures such as speed and accuracy, which show increased efficiency in the subject's processing of previously learned materials. The technique has been applied to objects and scene recognition as well as faces. EMMA, which stems from a theory-driven model of memory and adaptive function, appears to be promising. Published levels of correct classification across studies (grand mean = 88.1 percent) are on a par with results from standard polygraphs. More work is needed on the level of positive and negative predictive power across various samples of individuals. In addition, the methodology itself is somewhat constraining because it requires a specific type of knowledge on the part of the subject and a specific set of stimuli.

Specificity of Psychological States

The specificity of a psychological state should be reflected in the specificity of the neurophysiological index created for it. The neurophysiological index for a more general or superordinate psychological state is likely to be more easily validated than the corresponding index for a more specific psychological state. Deception in everyday matters is not as general a psychological state as information processing or fear or anxiety, but it is not as specific as lying about something as portentous as, say terrorism. Developers of new technologies must avoid making the same type of error. Turning to measurement of CNS response to deception (may represent) an attempt to develop an appropriate level of analysis for deception.

Reconsideration of Base Rates

The challenge posed by base rates can be overcome by applying signal detection theory, as mentioned above. Here is a substantive example. Assume that deception has a base rate of 1 in 1,000, and an index that is 90 percent accurate and that 10,000 individuals are being screened using the index. This assumed base rate is probably high if scientists are attempting to identify spies or terrorists in organizations as large as the military or in the populations of individuals on a given day traveling by air to or within the United States. As Table 2-1 from a report on the polygraph and lie detection illustrates (NRC, 2003), 1,598 people, or 99.5 percent of those who failed the screen and were (incorrectly) identified as spies or terrorists, would be false positives and 2 people (20 percent of the actual spies) who passed the screen and were identified as nonspies or nonterrorists would be false negatives. Only 8 (0.5 percent) of the people who failed the screen would actually be spies or terrorists and therefore true positives.

If the detection threshold is lowered to reduce the number of false positives, as Table 2-2 from the NRC report illustrates, the number of spies or terrorists who passed the screen (false negatives) would increase. In this case, 8 people (80 percent) of the spies or terrorists would have passed the screen. This example

TABLE 2-1 Rates of False Positives and False Negatives from Polygraph Examinations

Test Result	Subject's True Identity		
	Spy	Nonspy	Total
Fail	8	1,598	1,606
Pass	2	8,392	8,394
TOTAL	10	9,990	10,000

SOURCE: Adapted from NRC (2003).

TABLE 2-2 Increase in the Number of Spies or Terrorists Who Passed the Screen (False Negatives)

Test Result	Subject's True Identity		
	Spy	Nonspy	Total
Fail	2	39	41
Pass	8	9,951	9,959
TOTAL	10	9,990	10,000

SOURCE: Adapted from NRC (2003).

emphasizes the importance of a highly accurate test when testing large numbers of people for low-base-rate events, and calls attention to the care that must be taken in using the information when a less accurate test is involved.

These statistics make evident an important conclusion. When looking for targets in settings with a low base rate, such as screenings for terrorists at airports, achieving high confidence in a positive detection requires using a technology with an extremely high discriminating capacity on the order of that associated with HIV testing or the even more accurate DNA testing. If such a level of accuracy cannot be achieved using the test technology alone, further information that additionally differentiates true targets, and is external to the test technology, needs to be obtained and brought to bear.

Finding 2-2. The committee recognizes the IC's strong interest in improving its ability to detect deception. Consistent with the 2003 NRC study *The Polygraph and Lie Detection*, the committee uniformly agreed that, to date, insufficient, high-quality research has been conducted to provide empirical support for the use of any single neurophysiological technology, including functional neuroimaging, to detect deception.

Opinions differed within the committee concerning the near-term contribution of functional neuroimaging to the development of a system to detect deception in a practical or forensic sense. Committee members who conduct neuroimaging research largely agreed that studies published to date are promising and that further research is needed on the potential for neuroimaging to provide a more accurate method to determine deception. Importantly, human institutional review board standards require, at a minimum, that individuals not be put at any greater risk than they would be in their normal everyday lives. The committee believes that certain situations would allow such testing under "normal risk" situations; although the committee strongly endorses the necessity of realistic, but ethical, research in this area, it does not specify the nature of that research in this report.

Recommendation 2-1. The committee recommends further research on multi-modal methodological approaches for detecting and measuring neurophysiological indicators of psychological states and intentions. This research should combine multiple measures and assessment technologies, such as imaging techniques and the recording of electrophysiological, biochemical, and pharmacological responses. Resources invested in further cognitive neuroscience research should support programs of research based on scientific principles and that avoid the inferential biases inherent in previous research in polygraphy.

NEUROPSYCHOPHARMACOLOGY

Overview

Drugs and other mind-altering chemicals can influence all aspects of human psychology, including cognition, emotion, motivation, and performance. For known drugs, predictions of the type, onset, magnitude, and/or duration of effects in individuals or groups can be limited by incomplete knowledge of the interacting processes that govern drug effects. Clinical, field, and research experience reveals that drug effects in individual humans arise from interactions of multiple factors, including (but not limited to) the drug itself; its dose and route of use; the demand characteristics of the current situation; and the individual's health, physiology, and experience with drugs and performance demands. Attempts to predict the effects of new drugs are hampered by the possible surprise in structure, targets, delivery, mechanisms of action, interactions with other drugs, and varying performance conditions.

In the following discussion the committee uses the term "drug" to refer to any chemical agent with the capacity to alter human affect, cognition, motivation, or performance. Agents that can do this include not only pharmaceutical drugs for preventing, treating, or mitigating disease symptoms, but also foods, hormones, intoxicants, nutrients, plants, poisons, supplements, toxins, and so on. The porous boundaries among these classifications is exemplified by botulinum toxin type A, available by prescription as Botox. The actions and effects of drugs may change with long-term use or under altered conditions; may interact with medical, occupational, physical and psychological conditions; may affect individuals differently; and may affect human functions other than psychology. Effects may be perceived as beneficial, harmful, or neutral, and such perceptions may change with conditions.

Most discussions of drugs and their effects are organized along the lines of current models of brain and nervous system functioning. This method of organization can help to identify likely effects of known drugs but probably should not be used to identify potential dual-use threats. Changes in models of brain function may create new and surprising ideas about how, when, where, or why drugs produce their effects; about what those effects are; about the kinds of chemicals that function as drugs to alter human functioning; and about ways to enhance, minimize, or counteract drug effects. It is particularly important to realize that the drugs that changed psychiatry in the mid-twentieth century were not predicted by many pharmacological or psychological models of their time, perhaps especially in the United States (Swazey, 1974). Rather, the brief history of neuropsychopharmacology illustrates how the expectations of a particular cultural, medical, and research climate may cause a failure to predict new drugs, new ways of using drugs, or new drug effects. Recent advances in neuropsychopharmacology that have the potential to be "game changers" include a much improved knowledge of brain function and delivery systems such as are enabled by nanotechnology that would allow substances to cross the blood-brain barrier.

Many current psychotherapeutic drugs—that is, drugs used in treatment and management of psychiatric disorders—and their likely mechanisms of action were not anticipated by prior research or theory (Barrett, 2007). Classic examples of psychotherapeutic drugs with unexpected mechanisms of action and/or unanticipated effects, and called to attention by alert clinicians, include lithium, chlorpromazine, monoamine oxidase (MAO) inhibitors, and tricyclic antidepressants (Cade, 1949; Jarvik, 1970; Swazey, 1974). Another unexpected discovery was lead poisoning, which had long-lasting psychological effects in the employees of a workshop where batteries were made (Hamilton, 1915; International Labour Office, 1934). These examples suggest that new drugs with marked effects on critical psychological functions are "black swans," unanticipated events with effects that could not have been predicted, that may fail to be observed when they happen, or that have large, long-lasting consequences that go unrecognized (Taleb, 2007a,b).[4]

One modern drug with psychological effects that were not predicted by initial descriptions of its clinical pharmacology is ketamine. Developed in the private sector as an anesthetic, then discovered in clinical use to have hallucinogenic effects and co-opted into the club drug scene as Special K, it is now under investigation in the public and private sectors as a rapidly acting antidepressant and for the treatment of chronic pain; the use of ketamine as a rapid acting antidepressant remains unreplicated and provocative. Other such drugs are opioid antagonists as a treatment for alcoholism and cannabinoids. These examples suggest that current models of neuropsychopharmacological effect account post hoc for psychological effects of drugs and may have poor predictive ability.

In spite of the difficulty of predicting their psychological effects, psychotherapeutic drugs have proven to have greater clinical effectiveness than many other treatments. This has had important consequences for medical and cultural expectations about drugs. First, the discovery and clinical use of drugs for treatment and management of psychiatric disease have had far-reaching effects on research

---

[4]The term "black swan" as defined by Taleb (2007a,b) is an accepted term in the IC for unanticipated consequences. It should be noted that Taleb's "black swan" is not related to the older term "white crow" that implies sufficiency to disprove a hypothesis.

and practice in psychiatry, psychology, cognitive science, and other mental health and behavioral sciences. Demonstration that particular drugs could effectively treat psychiatric illnesses suggested that such illnesses were treatable much like other illnesses and promoted the medicalization of psychiatry. Equally important, the clinical usefulness of the earliest such drugs provided insight into the brain mechanisms that mediate the drugs' therapeutic efficacy and created opportunities for research to understand the chemical and biological bases of their effects. The critical linkage between drug effects and discoveries of brain receptors for neurotransmitters and other endogenous brain chemicals enabled the development of drugs with fewer side effects and more focused activity as well as a few truly new drugs that could target newly discovered chemical systems in the brain.

The appearance of clinically useful brain drugs occurred as the field of neuroscience coalesced so that medical and behavioral researchers could explore how biology manifests itself in behavior (Barrett, 2007; Dinges, 2007). One marker of the importance of the emerging field of neuroscience is the growth in attendance at the annual meeting of the premier professional association in the field, the Society for Neuroscience, from 1,396 in 1971 to 34,815 in 2005 (Society for Neuroscience, 2007).[5] Discoveries in neuroscience can be exploited to create new cellular or subcellular targets for drugs, new drug delivery systems, and new strategies to direct or control drug effects and achieve desired psychological effects. Novel classes of drugs approved by the Food and Drug Administration (FDA) illustrate the potential surprises of research, including drugs for erectile dysfunction, which arose from chemicals that were targeted at treatment of angina but failed to increase cardiac blood flow while unexpectedly increasing blood flow to the penis, and sleep-inducing drugs that exploit the roles of gamma aminobutyric acid (GABA) and melatonin receptors in brain sleep systems. Recent news stories on topics ranging from brain systems and drugs for memory enhancement (Rovner, 2007; Foer, 2007), appetite control (Bentivoglio and Kristensson, 2007), and sleep drugs (Saul, 2007) reflect the intense public, academic, and commercial interest in neuropsychopharmacology.

This interpretation of neuroscience research carries the additional implication that drugs can achieve or modulate not only abnormal, diseased, or disordered psychology but also normal, healthy, or optimal function. Development and utilization of drugs to treat psychiatric disorders have been accompanied by important changes in expectations of physicians, consumers, and policy makers about how drugs can and should be used (Barrett, 2007; Chatterjee, 2007; Kelly, 2007). These changes include expectations about the duration of a drug's use by an individual and who drives the choice of whether, when, and which drugs to use; opinions on personal drug use; and ideas about which human functions can, or should, be modulated by drug use. It may be particularly important that many

---

[5]See http://www.sfn.org/index.cfm?pagename=annualMeeting_statistics&section=annualMeeting. Last accessed December 17, 2007.

current prescription drugs, and possibly the majority of current prescription drugs with primarily psychological effects, are used widely off-label.[6] Such off-label use and the possibility of important placebo and nocebo effects (Lasagna et al., 1954, Beecher, 1955; Olshansky, 2007) cannot but open analysts' eyes to the probability that drugs have heretofore undiscovered effects.

Drugs that are described and marketed as having disease-specific or diagnosis-specific effects are quite capable of producing striking psychological effects in individuals who do not suffer from the condition identified with the drug's descriptive name or clinical indication. These psychological effects may or may not be similar to the effects in individuals with medical conditions for which the drugs are prescribed. Recent examples discussed in the public press include use of antipsychotic drugs for individuals without psychosis, beta-blockers to modulate performance anxiety in concert musicians, and steroids to enhance athletic performance. Other emerging changes in how drugs are prescribed and used include increased incidences of polypharmacy, of consumer decisions about whether and when to use drugs (as illustrated by erectile dysfunction drugs and Botox), and of consumer decisions to seek out and use available drugs for multiple effects. For example, the use of certain prescription drugs as study aids is not uncommon (White et al., 2006). Of 1,025 U.S. college students surveyed, 16.2 percent reported such use of prescription stimulants. Ninety percent of this group did not hold a legitimate prescription for stimulant drugs; 96 percent of them used Ritalin to improve attention, improve ability to participate in partying, reduce hyperactivity, and improve grades; and 15.5 percent reported using Ritalin at least two or three times per week.

Addiction and substance (or drug) abuse presents another area of change. The demarcation between abused drugs and medicines is situation dependent, as demonstrated by recent experience with OxyContin, by nicotine in over-the-counter smoking cessation aids, and by college-student exploitation of prescription stimulants. The illicit market not only provides incentives for novel drugs, manufacturing processes, and delivery systems but also poses novel risks. These factors are illustrated by episodes such as the appearance of permanent symptoms of Parkinson's disease in opiate addicts who used the illicitly manufactured 1-methyl-4-phenyl-1,2,3,6-tetrahydropyridine (MPTP), a neurotoxin probably produced by improper chemical conditions in illicit manufacture of meperidine, a synthetic opioid (Langston, 1995). The incentives provided by the illicit market are also exemplified by recent U.S. experience with methamphetamine labs and by the emergence of crack cocaine (smoked, minimal manufacturing danger, sold in small quantities) to challenge freebase cocaine (smoked, risks of explosion during manufacture), both of which challenged powdered cocaine (snorted or injected, sold in large quantities) (Kleiman, 1992; Musto, 1987). Epidemio-

---

[6]Under current FDA guidelines, manufacturers are prohibited from marketing approved drugs for off-label use.

logical and clinical research on the natural history of drug abuse also provides information about the long-term effects (often) high doses of at least a subset of performance-altering drugs, which may alert analysts to dual-use possibilities. The same may be true of patterns of drug use in highly competitive industries or markets, such as the steroids, stimulants, and endurance-altering drugs used by athletes or the stimulants used by floor traders.

Cognition Enhancers

One specific area of neuropsychopharmacology that may be of considerable importance is that of cognition enhancement. Cognition enhancers can be broadly defined as drugs or other agents that have the potential to improve human functions such as attention, learning, and memory (Sarter, 2006; Sahakian and Morein-Samir, 2007 and accompanying online discussion at http://network. nature.com/forums/naturenewsandopinion/). Considerable research investment in the United States and other countries is directed to the discovery and development of pharmacological cognition enhancers. Often, these agents target declines in memory and cognition linked to age, dementia, or neuropsychiatric or neurological disease. It is likely, however, that agents developed for prevention or treatment of disease will alter brain processes in normal individuals. Additionally, agents already in wide medical or social use are known to alter memory and cognition, sometimes by mechanisms shared with disease-related agents and sometimes by mechanisms not so clearly linked to age or pathology. Examples of widely used agents with known or suspected ability to alter and perhaps enhance certain components of human cognition and/or performance include caffeine (found in coffee, tea, soda), nicotine (tobacco products), tacrine (energy drinks), amphetamines and methylphenidate (attention deficit hyperactivity disorder medications and certain abused drugs), propranolol (certain beta-blockers), dextroamphetamine, and modafinil.

A fairly wide range of neuropharmacological or chemical systems have been suggested as possible sources for cognition or performance enhancers (e.g., Sarter, 2006). This expanding list is illustrative of the wide range of brain processes suspected of having potential to enhance normal and/or disordered cognition. Conversely, opposite changes or disruption in such systems might disrupt cognition and/or performance. Specifically, if agonists of a particular system enhance cognition, it is mechanistically plausible that antagonists might disrupt cognition; conversely, if antagonists of a particular neurotransmitter enhance, its agonists might disrupt. Examples of the former might include dopamine agonists, which enhance attention, and dopamine antagonists, which disrupt it; examples of the latter might include the suspected cognitive enhancing effects of cannabinoid antagonists and the disrupting effects of agonists like THC.

Three areas of research in behavioral pharmacology have particular importance for analysis of enhancement and/or disruption of cognition and performance. One identifies the boundaries or limitations of cognition enhancement. Many current models of cognition incorporate ideas of processing resources and their limitations. It is an open question as to whether drug-induced enhancements in one area of cognition have a cost in other areas. Stimulant drugs are known to have rate-dependent effects, such that the same exposure regimen may enhance attentional processes that are initially occurring with low frequency but simultaneously decrease attentional processes that are occurring at high frequency (Dews and Wenger, 1977), which could result in unwanted performance decrements. A cognition enhancer that optimizes performance under a taxing attention condition might not improve performance of a task with lower attention demands (Robbins, 2005) and in fact might disrupt it. As another example, drugs that enhance working memory capacity or operation may impair capacity to simultaneously filter distractors; this could increase false alarms in a detection operation (Lavie, 2005). Public recognition that modafinil, which promotes wakefulness and increases alertness, can have small but valuable cognitive effects is an example of a change that creates opportunities for public discussion of the risks and benefits of potential cognitive enhancers.

A second relevant area of behavioral pharmacology involves efforts to identify which specific neurochemical changes actually covary with cognitive processes. Studies of neurochemistry in cholinergic brain systems, for example, suggest that drug-induced changes in neurotransmitter release activated by attentional processes are vitally different from drug-induced changes in basal release (Sarter and Bruno, 1994; Kozak et al., 2006).

A third, and related, area is research to identify agents that produce specific kinds of cognitive enhancements rather than broadly acting agents (Rovner, 2007). Additionally, the full range of effects of potential cognition- or performance-enhancing drugs warrants attention. For example, stimulants such as amphetamine can increase attention and concentration, but they also exert cardiovascular effects that can be exacerbated by physical exertion and heat, and with prolonged or high dose use, they carry risks of addiction and paranoia.

Implications for Agents That May Act to Change or Disrupt Various Aspects of Human Psychology

There is currently a widely recognized "translational gap" between preclinical research, clinical research, and development of cognition enhancers, perhaps best articulated in the area of schizophrenia (Hagan and Jones, 2005; Floresco et al., 2005). Similar translational gaps exist in most, if not all, areas of neuropsychopharmacology. Examples of recognized roadblocks to new therapeutic entities include the need for improved clinical models, the rudimentary knowledge of brain neurochemistry and function, the paucity of models to predict side effects, and poor understanding of brain diseases and disorders. One recommendation for closing these translational gaps is to improve the predictive power of animal models so that they map onto operationally defined domains of affective, cognitive, and motivational processes (Robbins, 1998; Sarter, 2006; Barrett, 2007). The neuronal bases of cognitive function are poorly understood, and most animal models that are used to identify potentially useful therapeutics are not based on molecular- or systems-level understanding of brain processes or on functional understanding of human cognition and behavior. Improved animal models for human psychopathology (depression, anxiety, memory decline, cognitive failure) and for normal functioning (learning, affect, motivation, performance) could permit development of novel drugs and/or drugs that can be targeted to effect human cognition and performance. While animal models are useful, many effects on cognitive dimensions cannot really be tested on rats or mice.

The discovery of the probable role of the hypocretins (also called orexins) in human narcolepsy shows that once the chemistry is known and the market drivers are in place, a drug can be developed rapidly. Symptoms of narcolepsy are currently managed with amphetamine-like CNS stimulants or modafinil (for excessive daytime sleepiness) and antidepressants or sodium oxylate (for cataplexy), but none of these treatments are based on an understanding of how brain chemistry is dysregulated in affected individuals. Recent research, which arose from the discovery of narcolepsy genes in animal models, suggests that a deficiency of hypocretin/orexim is responsible for about 90 percent of human narcolepsy-cataplexy cases (Nishino, 2007a,b). This finding led directly to development of new diagnostic tests for narcolepsy and has led to the search for new therapeutic drugs for narcolepsy caused by a deficiency of hypocretin/orexim. Additionally, novel small-molecule hypocretin/orexim receptor antagonists that can be used to inhibit feeding have been identified.

Finding 2-3. Neurochemical systems modulate, and can be used to control, a wide range of human psychology. The number of neuropsychopharmacological drugs increased dramatically after the mid-1900s, along with their availability, and emerging technologies may improve the ability to harness drug effects or to produce targeted changes in human psychology. Cognitive neuroscientists do not have specific understanding of how most drugs produce their effects. Basic research in the public or private sectors that identifies the specific mechanisms of disease and of drug effects might enable rapid development of new drugs. New drugs may have unrecognized effects that emerge owing to variation in individuals, settings, or performance demands.

Nanotechnology in Medicine

In addition to bringing new drug entities or new uses for existing entities, emerging technologies might allow new pathways for drug delivery. Some observers say it is likely that the paradigm of the pharmaceutical industry will change, from "discovering" drugs by screening many compounds to the purposeful engineering of desired molecules.

Richard Feynman famously said, "There's plenty of room at the bottom," in a lecture in which he outlined the principle of manipulating individual atoms using larger machines to manufacture increasingly smaller machines (Feynman, 1959). Nanotechnology is a rapidly expanding, multidisciplinary field that applies engineering and manufacturing principles at a molecular level. It can be roughly divided into categories that include nanobiotechnology, biological microelectromechanical systems, microfluidics, biosensors, microarrays, and tissue microengineering (Gourley, 2005). In some sense nanotechnology is intuitive, since everything in nature is built upward from the atomic level in order to define limits and structures (Emerich and Thanos, 2006). Understanding and developing nanotechnology, therefore, depends on understanding these limits and pushing against them.

Nanomedicine (the development of effective clinical treatments based on nanotechnology) has had some successes (Freitas, 1999) and depends on several overlapping molecular technologies. These new but progressing technologies include (1) the construction of nanoscale-sized structures for diagnostics, biosensors, and local drug delivery; (2) genomics, proteomics, and nanoengineered microbes; and (3) the creation of molecular machines capable of identifying and eliminating host pathogens by replacing and repairing cells and cellular components in vivo (Emerich and Thanos, 2006). Of particular importance may be nanotechnologies that allow delivery of drugs across the blood-brain barrier in ways now impossible.

Nanotechnology for Drug Delivery

In the last decade nanotechnology and nanofabrication have significantly impacted the field of drug delivery (Emerich and Thanos, 2006). The continued development of these technologies will probably occur in conjunction with the development of pharmaceuticals targeted at the brain (Ellis-Behnke et al., 2007; Jain, 2007; Koo et al., 2006; Silva, 2006, 2007; Suri et al., 2007; Teixido and Giralt, 2008). The development of such neuropharmaceutical combinations is of great interest to the Department of Defense. Guided by the statement of task, the committee outlines in the following paragraphs nanotechnologies that may contribute to advances in the delivery of CNS drugs.

Techniques have shifted from microfabrication and micromachining (e.g., the osmotic pump) to designs ranging from secondary constructs at the nanometer scale (e.g., microspheres). The engineering of nano delivery systems for small molecules, proteins, and DNA has led to the emergence of entirely new and previously unpredicted fields. Formulation science has linked up with computer technology to create a controlled-release microchip capable of infinite modulation that would allow for the greatly improved controlled release of pharmaceutical agents (Santini et al., 1999; Grayson et al., 2003; Maloney et al., 2005; Prescott et al., 2006). Tissue engineering applications have also moved toward the development and implementation of nanometer-sized components. The creation of artificial cells with appropriate physiologic properties may provide a better understanding of normal physiological processes. Transfection systems on the nanoscale for genetic manipulation and gene delivery are being tailored using different polymers.

Nanotechnology is opening new therapeutic opportunities for agents that could not be used effectively as conventional drug formulations owing to their poor bioavailability or drug instability (Santini et al., 1999). Microsphere formulations are used to protect agents susceptible to degradation or denaturation while prolonging their duration of action by increasing systemic exposure or retention of the formulation (Hillyer and Albrecht, 2001; Hussain et al., 2001; Torche et al., 2000; Van Der Lubben et al., 2001; Varde and Pack, 2004). Nanoparticles are able to cross membrane barriers, particularly in the absorptive epithelium of the small intestine (Hillyer and Albrecht, 2001) and are being used to deliver small molecules, proteins, and other therapeutics (Dunning et al., 2004; Hamaguchi et al., 2005; Koushik et al., 2004; Panyam and Labhasetwar, 2003; Silva, 2006; Weissleder et al., 2005). Biodegradable nanospheres enhance bioavailability through uptake, followed by degradation and disappearance of the vehicle from the system.

Integration of controlled-release drug reservoirs with microchips (Santini et al., 1999) provides unlimited potential for modulating drug release. Nanotubes that have large relative internal volumes also can be functionalized on the inside surface (Martin and Kohli, 2003). One fabrication technique used self-assembling lipid microtubes to deliver testosterone in rats (Goldstein et al., 2001). Testosterone was covalently bound with an ester linkage to a glutamide core lipid, forming nanotubes that possessed an in vivo biphasic release profile characterized by an initial burst followed by a more sustained release. Another method of fabrication involves synthesizing carbon nanotubes using fullerene. These nanotubes range from one nanometer to tens of nanometers in diameter and are from several to hundreds of microns long. Drugs can be covalently attached to functional groups on the external surface of the nanotubes (Chen et al., 2001). Another drug delivery approach uses nanoshells or dielectric-metal (gold-coated silica) nanospheres. When embedded in a drug-containing polymer and then injected into the body, these nanoshells accumulate near tumor cells. When heated with an infrared laser, the polymer melts, releasing the drug at a specific site (Hirsch et al., 2005; Loo et al., 2005). This technology allows delivering drugs at very precise locations in the brain. Growing knowledge about the neural circuits underlying various functions will probably enhance the capacity to target specific effects with fewer side effects.

Improvements in drug-containing nanoparticles are already gaining regulatory approval. Abraxane, a nanoparticle form of albumin and paclitaxel,[7] elimi-

---

[7]For additional information, see http://www.cancer.gov. Last accessed on January 24, 2008.

nates the need for toxic solvents in earlier versions of paclitaxel (Taxol) and permits more of the drug to be administered. Similarly, a micellar nanoparticle formulation of paciltaxel (NK105) is being developed to reduce toxicity while enhancing antitumor activity (Hamaguchi et al., 2005). There is broad international interest in research on nanotechnology for drug delivery. Asia, in particular, is active in this area, as evidenced by the published literature (Bosi et al., 2000; Miyata and Yamakoshi, 1997; Chen et al., 2001; Tabata et al., 1997a,b; Tsao et al., 1999, 2001; Hamaguchi et al., 2005), and there is especially strong research in drug delivery to the brain and neuropeptides (Gao et al., 2007a,b).[8]

Finding 2-4. Technological advances will affect the types of neuropsychopharmacological drugs available and methods for drug delivery. For the IC, nanotechnologies that allow drugs to cross the blood-brain barrier, increase the precision of delivery, evade immune system defenses, evade metabolism, or prolong actions at cellular or downstream targets will be of particular importance. These technologies will increase the likelihood that various peptides, or other brain proteins, could ultimately be utilized as drugs. Development of antidotes or protective agents against various classes of drugs that could be used by an enemy force will also be important.

Neuropeptides and Behavior

Neuropeptides act as messengers in the brain, influencing many neurobehavioral functions (Strand, 1999). Their therapeutic use in humans has been hampered because they do not readily pass the blood-brain barrier (BBB) and they induce potent hormonelike side effects in the blood (Illum, 2000; Pardridge, 1999). To date, the results of intranasal administration testing have been mixed (Born et al., 2002; Heinrichs et al., 2003; Heinrichs et al., 2004; Merkus and van den Berg, 2007). However, nanotechnology may someday allow for quick pharmacological modifications of behaviors. Box 2-2 provides an overview of the function of the BBB.

One neuropeptide of interest is oxytocin, which—in addition to its well-known functions in milk letdown and childbirth—has a central role in positive social behavioral interactions and can increase trust behavior in human experimental subjects. Oxytocin receptors are distributed in brain regions associated with certain behaviors (Huber et al., 2005; Landgraf and Neumann, 2004) such as pair bonding, maternal care, sexual behavior, and the ability to form normal social attachments (Carter, 1998; Carter et al., 2001; Heinrichs et al., 2002; Huber et al., 2005; Insel and Young, 2001; Pedersen, 1997; Uvnäs-Moberg, 1998; Young et al., 2001). Thus oxytocin permits animals to overcome their natural avoidance

---

[8]Psivida Ltd. of Australia and SkyePharma of Great Britain are two examples of international interest in this area of research. For additional information, see http://www.psivida.com/. Last accessed on April 10, 2008.

Box 2-2
The Blood-Brain Barrier as an Obstacle to the
Delivery of Therapeutics

The blood-brain barrier (BBB) remains an obstacle to the delivery of therapeutics to the brain.[a] It comprises an endothelial cell monolayer associated with pericytes and astrocytes. The BBB separates the blood from the cerebral parenchyma and prevents the penetration of drugs into the CNS. The BBB was first noticed by Paul Ehrlich in 1885 and later confirmed by Edwin Goldmann. It protects the brain from substances that can be neurotoxic in physiological concentrations—for example, potassium, glycine, and glutamate (Gururangan and Friedman, 2002). This physical barrier is characterized by tight intercellular junctions (zonulae occludens) (Brightman and Reese, 1969) and by the absence of fenestrations, both of which limit the penetration of therapeutic molecules. The deficiency in pinocytic vesicles and the high metabolic capacity of cerebral endothelial cells (Reese and Karnovsky, 1967) also help to limit the exchange of anticancer agents between the plasma and the CNS. Furthermore, the cerebral endothelium has a high level of ATP-binding cassette (ABC) transporters such as P-glycoprotein involved in drug efflux mechanisms (Golden and Pollack, 2003). Thus the BBB prevents the uptake of all large-molecule drugs and more than 98 percent of pharmaceutical small-molecule drugs. Only very small (<5 KD_a), lipid-soluble, electrically neutral molecules and weak bases are able to diffuse passively across the BBB (Abraham et al., 1994).

---

[a]For more information on nanotechnology for neuroscience, neuropeptides, and the blood-brain barrier, which is beyond the scope of this report, see Beduneau et al. (2006), Pardridge (1999, 2001), Emerich and Thanos (2006), and Strand (1999).

---

of proximity and facilitates approach behavior. Given that oxytocin is believed to promote social attachment and affiliation in nonhuman mammals, researchers have hypothesized it might also promote more social behaviors—such as trust—in humans (Kosfeld et al., 2005; Zak et al., 2007; Zak and Fakhar, 2006).

FUNCTIONAL NEUROIMAGING

Introduction

Broadly defined, functional neuroimaging is the use of neuroimaging technology to measure aspects of brain function, often with the goal of understanding the relationship between regional brain activity and specific tasks, stimuli, cognition, behaviors or neural processes. Common technologies for functional neuroimaging include multichannel electroencephalography (EEG), magneto-encephalography (MEG), positron emission tomography (PET), functional magnetic resonance imaging (fMRI), functional near-infrared spectroscopy (fNIRS), functional transcranial Doppler sonography (fTCDS), and magnetic resonance spectroscopy (MRS). EEG and MEG measure localized electrical or magnetic fluctuations in neuronal activity. PET, fMRI, fNIRS, and fTCDS can measure localized changes in cerebral blood flow related to neural activity. PET and MRS can measure regional modulation of brain metabolism and neurochemistry in response to neural activity or processes. These functional neuroimaging technologies are complementary, and each offers a different window onto complex neural processes. Because of this complementarity, multimodal imaging is an emerging area of great interest for research, clinical, commercial, and defense applications.

Neuroimaging technologies are likely to play an important role in endeavors to enhance cognition as well as affect and motivation over the next two decades. Predictions about future applications of technology are always speculative, but if the issues discussed above come to fruition this emergent technology might provide insight into the following areas, and others, of direct relevance to national defense: the acquisition of intelligence from captured unlawful combatants, enhanced training techniques, augmented cognition and memory enhancement of soldiers and intelligence operatives, the screening of terrorism suspects at checkpoints or ports of entry where there are no constitutional protections (i.e., airports), and soldier-machine interface devices such as are used in remotely piloted vehicles and prosthetics. Indeed, science is already beginning to see contributions of this field to clinical and battlefield medicine.

Over the next two decades, good brain-computer interfaces (BCIs) are likely to be a great of interest to the gaming industry as well as to the rehabilitation, medical, and military sectors, and neuroimaging and neurophysiology will play a central role in those endeavors. BCIs are likely to be used to enhance several areas of cognition, including memory, concentration, and emotional intelligence, among others. Indeed, this has been a focus of the Defense Advance Research Projects Agency's (DARPA's) Augmented Cognition program for several years. Brain prosthetics could become the new input-output devices for memory systems, allowing efficient searching and encyclopedic access to information. Sandberg and Bostrom suggest BCIs may improve better concentration by reducing working memory load and exploiting the broad attention abilities of the visual system.

Similarly, DARPA has been working on EEG and fNIRS-based BCIs that use the human visual system as the input device to a computer system to increase the speed of data processing in visual search mode. The idea is that although current technological capacities with computer vision are not even close to the speed and sophistication of the human eye, there is a lag time between the visual mental process and a motor output to the computer system. By using EEG or fNIRS to directly measure the brain's response when it detects a target, the search process can occur more quickly than with an operator's motor response. Given the current level of miniaturization of computer memory, a wearable computer with an efficient brain-based input/output device (a "mental mouse") and an efficient search strategy could allow access to huge amounts of stored data in milliseconds, effectively augmenting the user's long-term memory. Such devices could allow military troops to access visual maps and intelligence when they approach a new area or to access medical information in the field.

Sandberg and Bostrom suggest that wearable computers could also enhance emotional intelligence—that is, the ability to perceive emotions in others and respond appropriately. Such capabilities could be useful for gathering intelligence. The current prototype system was designed to help people who have difficulty in accurately assessing the emotions of other people—for example, children with Asperger syndrome—by improving their ability to interact (El Kaliouby and Robinson, 2005). The system consists of a camera to record the facial expressions of a conversational partner, facial and emotion processing software that estimates the most likely emotional state, a readout that displays a cartoon of the emotion, and suggestions for a proper response. Such systems could also help a participant in a high-stakes negotiation or interview to gauge more accurately the emotional intentions of his or her counterpart (see, for example, Ekman and O'Sullivan, 2006). Indeed, Ekman and Mark Frank (Frank and Ekman, 2004), along with others at DARPA, have been using computer-aided analysis of facial responses based on Ekman's theories to study at-a-distance measures of deception.

Owing to their awkward size and shape and their cost, some technologies such as MEG and MRI/fMRI are likely to take a backseat in enabling cognitive enhancement, providing the underlying neuroscience upon which more fieldable technologies, such as EEG and fNIRS, can be based. It is, for example, unlikely that brain–computer interfaces based on fMRI could be loaded onto jets or spaceships in the next two decades, whereas an EEG or fNIRS-based system could very well be so deployed in that timeframe. However, the information about cognitive, affective, and motivational states that accrues from these various kinds of neuroimaging is likely to play a key role in the use of technology-based systems to enhance performance.

Another example is the use of transcranial magnetic stimulation (TMS) to facilitate neural changes that have been identified through neuroimaging. TMS is a noninvasive way to excite neurons in the brain: rapidly changing magnetic fields (electromagnetic induction) are used to induce weak electric currents in neural tissue, allowing the brain to be activated from outside with minimal discomfort. One alternative to using pharmacological agents to influence neural function is to use electrical stimulation such as TMS to excite the neuromodulatory centers that control plasticity. Experiments in the monkey have shown that electrical stimulation can result in faster cortical reorganization. In their review, Sandberg and Bostrom cite evidence that TMS can increase or decrease the excitability of the cortex, in turn changing its level of plasticity. TMS has been used to facilitate the learning of a procedural memory task by stimulating the motor cortex. Sandberg and Bostrom suggest TMS has succeeded in facilitating working memory, classification, learning motor skills such as finger tapping sequences, coordinating visuomotor tasks, and consolidating declarative memory during sleep.

Because TMS is noninvasive and able to improve performance on a variety of cognitive tasks, Sandberg and Bostrom suggest that it could be a very versatile tool for cognitive enhancement. One limitation is the short duration of its effect (minutes to an hour after stimulation), although some results suggest that coupling TMS with pharmacological manipulations of the dopaminergic system could facilitate long-term consolidation or longer effects TMS (Nitsche et al., 2006). It is worthwhile reminding the reader that the considerable interindividual variability in responses to TMS might require individual tuning of dosage, placement, and so on. Neuroimaging tools such as MRI, fMRI, or fNIRS could play a role in providing precise localization for such technology integrations.These functional neuroimaging technologies, some mature, others emergent, are commonplace in research and clinical environments and are having an impact on defense policy decisions (Peters et al., 2008). Recent advances and developments allow for functional neuroimaging capability with real-time or near-real-time data acquisition and analysis that is becoming cheaper, portable, and more user friendly. Continued refinement of these technologies is likely to lead to increased dissemination of this technology, with applications expanding well beyond the current primary fields of neuroscience research and clinical medicine. Areas where the application of advanced functional neuroimaging technology likely are business (marketing, economics, human resources), human performance, risk assessment, the field of law, and the military, all of them having great relevance to national policy and defense issues. Progress continues to be made in both functional neuroimaging and neurophysiological methods toward the holy grail of neuroimaging, namely, millisecond-level temporal resolution with precise spatial localization. No current technology affords both high temporal resolution and high spatial resolution with access to the full brain. The strengths and limitations of each technology are briefly described below.

Electroencephalography

The oldest device used to assess brain function in real time is the electroencephalograph. Many years ago it became known that electrical activity in the brain could be recorded by placing electrodes on the surface of the scalp (Berger, 1929). Such recordings represent the summated electrical signal from nominally 50,000 local neurons. Early studies focused on the spontaneous rhythmic oscillations in voltage—frequency bands that tended to shift together with changing mental status, such as alpha waves, which have frequencies between 8 and 13 Hz. Early clinical EEG was used primarily to detect and diagnose epilepsy, but today, with advances in computer technology, informative new experimental paradigms and techniques are being developed. Electroencephalographic recordings are of two main types: continuous and discrete. Continuous recordings are the traditional multitrace waveforms recorded since EEGs began and activity is classified by the frequency of the dominant waveform (0-40 Hz) on any given channel, such as alpha waves. Discrete recordings are triggered by an event, such as an external flash of light, and then the next 1 to 4 seconds of activity are recorded. In discrete recordings, the "normal" EEG waves are considered background.

Discrete, or event-related, recordings were first described by Davis (1939), who noticed that event-related changes could be seen in an ongoing electroencephalogram event-related potentials (ERPs), currently the focus of electroencephalographic research, refer to the measurement of the brain's electrophysiological response to a particular stimulus. The brain's response to discrete stimuli are typically relatively small (a few microvolts) compared with the ongoing background EEG activity (approximately 50 mV), and multiple stimulus presentations are averaged to distinguish the response associated with the stimulus from the background activity. When the brain response is largely automatic and dictated by the physical properties of the stimulus (say, the loudness of a sound or the brightness of a light flash) it is called an evoked potential. Evoked potentials generally occur 15-100 ms after a stimulus is presented. Later responses, which occur as early as 150 ms after a stimulus, are thought to be influenced by cognitive processes and are referred to as ERPs.

Quantitative electroencephalography (QEEG) uses postrecording computer analysis to analyze the relationship between each of the electrodes placed at the scalp. The frequency composition, amplitude, and position of each electrode is compared to the same information taken from a database of individuals without any known neurological disorder. The resulting EEG brain maps are then analyzed with sophisticated statistical techniques to reveal patterns. The results of these analyses can be presented in graphical form as topographical displays of brain electrical activity. Applications include neurofeedback, or neurotherapy, and the identification of responses to medication for certain neurological and psychiatric disorders. Neurotherapy is an experimental technique that uses a QEEG brain map to analyze psychiatric problems from attention deficit disorder to depression to schizophrenia. Patients are then subjected to a conditioning protocol to "train" the "abnormal" brain activity toward a statistically more "normal" pattern of activity. Neurotherapy can reduce aberrant symptoms of many conditions (Fox et al., 2005).

Interpretation of a scalp electroencephalogram often involves speculation as to the location inside the brain of the source of the activity recorded (Brazier, 1949; Shaw and Roth, 1955). While there is substantial PET and fMRI literature on finding the neural sources of the functional network implicated in given mental tasks (Cabeza and Nyberg, 2000), PET and fMRI are temporally limited in their ability to probe discrete neural events. The source localization capability of EEG has been used to overcome this limitation and solve the inverse problem. Even though EEG offers millisecond-level time resolution, the signals measured at the scalp do not directly indicate the location of the neurons that are generating the activity. Although the sites at which the scalp potentials are measured at any given point in time are finite, an infinite number of source configurations could account for those measurements (Plonsey, 1963; Fender, 1987). Source localization involves mathematical attempts to solve the inverse problem by introducing a priori assumptions about the generation of the EEG (or MEG) signals. The better these assumptions are, the more trustworthy the source estimations will be, and several different models have been formulated and implemented in algorithms to reach the inverse solution, each using different mathematical, biophysical, statistical, anatomical, or functional constraints (for a recent review, see Michel et al., 2004). Technological advances in the field include noncontact electrodes that use high-gain preamplifiers to mitigate the effects of the high impedance caused by the lack of contact. This arrangement could allow the "application" of a large number of electrodes in a relatively short time, at the cost of a noisier signal. As these models and constraint estimates improve, there is promise for important future developments. EEG has several advantages over other functional neuroimaging techniques, including the relatively low cost of the technology (around $15 million). Also, a single technician can produce reliable recordings with unmatched temporal resolution measured in milliseconds. A number of other countries use high-density EEG with source localization.[9]

Positron Emission Tomography

The introduction of computed tomography (CT) by Sir Godfrey Hounsfield in 1973 (Petrik et al., 2006) dramatically changed the way scientists and physicians examined the brain. The development of PET (based on prior brain autoradiographic work) quickly followed, creating in vivo autoradiograms of brain function (Ter-Pogossian et al., 1975; Phelps et al., 1975) and introducing a new era of functional brain mapping. For an excellent historical review of PET and functional neuroimaging the reader is referred to Raichle (1998).

PET can be used to produce a three-dimensional image or map of functional processes in the brain. The system detects pairs of gamma rays emitted indirectly by a positron-emitting radioisotope, which is introduced into the body on a metabolically active molecule. Images of regional metabolic activity or blood flow are then reconstructed by computer analysis. Modern versions of PET scanners are combined with CT scanning and MRI scanning capability to coregister metabolic activity with high-resolution anatomic images of the brain, creating three-dimensional metabolic/anatomic overlays.

---

[9]In Cuba, some scientists are reportedly doing very accurate localization using high-density EEG arrays to locate tumors. Personal communication to committee member Scott Bunce from Roy John.

The radionuclides utilized in PET scanning typically have short half lives; carbon-11 (~20 min), nitrogen-13 (~10 min), oxygen-15 (123), and fluorine-18 (~110 min). They are incorporated into compounds such as glucose and water. These radiotracers distribute in the brain by following the metabolic pathways of their natural analogues or by binding with specificity to the receptor proteins for which they have affinity. Due to the short half lives of most radioisotopes, the radiotracers must be produced in a cyclotron and a certified medicinal radiochemistry laboratory co-located with the PET facility. Fluorine-18, with a half life long enough to allow commercial manufacture at an offsite location and transport to an imaging center daily, is an exception.

PET has gained widespread utility in clinical medicine, particularly in oncology, where it has become the favored imaging technology for the detection, staging, and monitoring of response to treatment for many neoplasms. Clinical PET is also used in neurology, psychiatry, cardiology, and pharmacology. There is continued widespread use of PET technology to study brain metabolism and receptor ligands. Limitations of PET include its relatively low temporal resolution; spatial resolution limited to approximately 5 mm; relatively expensive equipment; requirement for an injectable, short-lived positron-emitting radioisotope that is usually produced in a cyclotron; and limits on its use for repetitive longitudinal studies and studies in certain populations owing to its emission of ionizing radiation.

However, PET remains a powerful tool for functional neuroimaging, especially with the proliferation of PET/CT and PET/MRI scanners. PET's exquisite ability to elucidate specific receptor binding sites/activity within the brain and its ability to produce images of brain metabolism mean it is not likely to be supplanted by other neuroimaging technologies in the foreseeable future. Indeed molecular neuroimaging via PET is likely to show the most growth in functional neuroimaging research over the next decade (Hammound et al., 2007).

Functional Magnetic Resonance Imaging

MRI is widely accepted as the gold standard for anatomical neuroimaging. The most common form of functional MRI (fMRI) utilizes a blood-oxygenation-level-dependent (BOLD) contrast mechanism to distinguish areas of neural activity. Other methodologies for fMRI include dynamic contrast techniques and noncontrast techniques (e.g., arterial spin labeling). There has been explosive growth of fMRI research and clinical applications over the past decade, with research applications including brain mapping of task (motor and cognitive) dependent processes. MRI has also been employed for detection of deception, an application that has drawn the interest of various communities (ethics, defense, legal). Under controlled experimental conditions with cooperative subjects, this technology has shown initial promise (Abe et al., 2006, 2007; Mohamed et al., 2006; Davatzikos et al., 2005; Kozel et al., 2004a,b, 2005; Langleben et al., 2002,

2005; Lee et al., 2002, 2005; Nuñez et al., 2005; Phan et al., 2005a; Ganis et al., 2003; Spence et al., 2001).

Real-time data acquisition (single-trial fMRI) and near-real-time data analysis (hundreds of milliseconds delay) of complex cognitive tasks have been demonstrated and will expand the applications areas of relevance to the research, clinical, and defense communities (Posse et al., 2003; Phan et al., 2004). Real-time fMRI has been utilized to demonstrate the voluntary suppression of affective state, suggesting that it may provide insight into complex cognitive processes (Phan et al., 2005b). Whether these findings can be generalized to nonexperimental settings remains to be determined. fMRI has many advantages over other functional imaging techniques, including high spatial resolution of the activation patterns (measured in millimeters); temporal resolution (measured in a few seconds); no known risk factors in healthy subjects;[10] and, recently near-real-time analysis. Its key disadvantages include its relatively high cost; problems with data interpretation if the subject moves a few millimeters; a user-unfriendly scanning environment (noisy, small enclosed space); and the requirement for large superconducting magnets.

Recent advances in neuroimaging technology, including high-field (3 tesla) and ultrahigh-field (7 tesla) magnetic resonance techniques for MRI, fMRI and MRS, real-time acquisition/processing, and parallel imaging, offer the potential for significant advances in spatial and temporal resolution for structural, functional and neurochemical imaging. In other words, MRI-based imaging technologies are providing faster and more detailed pictures of the human brain and brain function than ever before. These and other related technologies are moving forward rapidly, driven by clinical and research demand, and over the next two decades there are likely to be continuing significant advances in this technology, with unique applications certain to emerge (Dickerson, 2007; Ladd, 2007; Nakada, 2007).

As shown in Table 2-3, a concerted effort at the national level in China to invest in research relating to high-field structural and functional fMRI has led to a network of coordinated laboratories and programs (Cao et al., 2006; Poo and Guo, 2007; Simon, 2007).[11]

Magnetic Resonance Spectroscopy

Magnetic resonance spectroscopy (MRS) provides a noninvasive window into brain chemistry. Research clinical applications include the ability to differentiate pathology (e.g., brain neoplasm) from normal or necrotic tissue (Moore,

---

[10]The main injuries during MRI are caused by the magnetic field being attracted by the ferrous (i.e., magnetic) substances within the body. Proper screening of subjects by attending personnel eliminates this risk.

[11]Personal communication between committee chair Christopher Green and Amy Kohl of Wayne State School of Medicine.

TABLE 2-3 Current Neuroimaging Research in the People's Republic of China

Name	Location	Machines	Known Use of Machines[a]
Xuanwu Hospital	Beijing	1.5 T, 3 T Siemens TRIO	Clinical and research; 14 articles published 2007
Beijing Friendship Hospital	Beijing	0.5 T Philips Gyroscan T5-NT	Clinical and research
Beijing MRI Center for Brain Research	Beijing	3 T Siemens TRIO	Research; 7 articles published 2007
Beijing MRI Center for Brain Research	Beijing	3 T Siemens Verio	Believed delivered October 2007 two units wide bore PET scanner insert
Tsinghua University	Beijing	Has access to low field, 1.5 T and 3 T	Research
Beijing Hospital	Beijing	1.5 T, 3 T Philips Achieva	Clinical and research; 8 articles published 2007
Beijing Jishuitan Hospital	Beijing	Unknown	Clinical and research
Institute of Biophysics	Beijing	1.5 T GE, 3 T Siemens TRIO	Research
Tian Tan Hospital	Beijing	Unknown	Clinical and research; 9 articles published 2007
An Zhen Hospital	Beijing	1.5 T Siemens Sonata	Clinical and research
China-Japan Friendship Hospital	Beijing	0.5 T	Clinical and research; 13 articles published 2007
Peking University First Hospital	Beijing	1.5 T GE and a 3 T GE Signa	Clinical and research; 9 articles published 2007
Peking Union Medical College Hospital	Beijing	Unknown	Clinical and research
Peking University Third Hospital	Beijing	1.5 T Siemens Magnetom	Clinical and research; 8 articles published 2007
Second Xiangya Hospital	Changsha	1.5 T GE	Clinical and research; 9 articles published 2007

continued

TABLE 2-3 Continued

Name	Location	Machines	Known Use of Machines[a]
Guilin Medical College	Guilin	1.5 T	Clinical and research
University of Science and Technology of China	Hefei	Unknown	Research
Shanghai Children's Medical Center	Shanghai	1.5 T	Clinical and research
Shanghai 9th People's Hospital	Shanghai	0.2 T Siemens Magnetom Open	Clinical and research
Xin Hua Hospital	Shanghai	0.5 T	Clinical and research; 5 articles published 2007
Renji Hospital	Shanghai	1.5 T Philips, 1.0 T Philips Gyroscan NT	Clinical and Research
Ruijin Hospital	Shanghai	1.5 T GE Signa	Clinical and research; 7 articles published 2007
MR Application Academy	Shanghai	Unknown	Training
Changhai Hospital	Shanghai	1.5 T Siemens Symphony	Clinical and research; 11 articles published 2007
Anhui Wu Jing Hospital	Shanghai	0.35 T Siemens C!	Unknown

[a]As of January 10, 2008.

1998); monitoring brain metabolism (glutamate, glucose levels); and monitoring neuropharmacologic treatment effects (neurotropic/neuroprotective medicines or psychoactive compounds) (Manji et al., 1999; Moore et al., 2000). While spatial resolution is on the order of 1 cc, this methodology has the potential to monitor neurochemical modulation in response to neural processes or neuropharmacologic intervention. Multiple studies have demonstrated the ability of MRS to detect biomarkers of complex neural processes, and rapid (<30 sec) neurochemical imaging becomes possible with high-field magnetic resonance technology (Phan et al., 2005c). Advances in MRS should be followed carefully because its complementarity with respect to the other functional neuroimaging technologies, particularly in the area of monitoring neuropharmacologic response, is likely to make it applicable for defense purposes. For example, as the ability to monitor neurochemistry in vivo and in near real time is developed with advanced high-field MRS and related technologies, the possibility arises of developing state-dependent neurochemical biomarkers for stress and anxiety as well as their pharmacologic modulation in a dose response fashion.

Magnetoelectroencephalography

Magnetoencephalography (MEG) is a completely noninvasive, nonhazardous technology for functional brain mapping, localizing and characterizing the electrical activity of the CNS by measuring the associated magnetic fields emanating from the brain. Every electrical current generates a magnetic field. However, unlike an electrical signal, magnetic fields are not distorted by traveling through the skull, and the source of the summated magnetic fields can be triangulated within a few millimeters. MEG provides functional mapping information on the working brain.

Modern MEG scanners use as many as 300 superconducting quantum interference device (SQUID)[12] detectors, allowing very fast acquisition and extremely high localization of the source of the electromagnetic signal. The information provided by MEG is entirely different from but complementary to the information provided by structural imaging techniques like CT or MR imaging. While MRI and CT provide excellent anatomical images, MEG measures correlates of neurological function. The advantages of MEG over fMRI and PET include the measurement of brain activity with higher temporal and spatial resolution. Its disadvantages include its greater cost than fMRI. It also requires a specialized technical team with broad expertise in the acquisition and processing of complex data and requires very precise positioning requirements.

Transcranial Ultrasonography

While transcranial ultrasonography operates on the same principle as the diagnostic ultrasound imaging of a fetus in utero, it is more difficult to obtain high-quality images of the brain because the propagation of sound waves is impaired by bone. However, the skull is thin enough in a few "monographic windows" (Duscheck and Schandry, 2003) to provide a path for the ultrasonic signal and can provide accurate real-time measurements of blood flow velocity. The transorbital window, located above the zygomatic arch (the "temple"), is used to image the posterior, anterior, and medial cerebral arteries along with a few of the branches that provide blood flow to specific areas of the brain.

---

[12]SQUID: Superconducting Quantum Interference Device, supercooled electronic component designed to detect extremely small changes in magnetic fields.

Although both rely on blood flow, sonography is very different from fMRI, which measures blood oxygenation level changes with a spatial resolution of a couple of millimeters. In functional transcranial doppler sonography (fTDS), the spatial resolution is determined by the volume of the brain supplied with blood by the vessel under study. These areas can be quite large, making the spatial resolution of fTDS extremely limited. Changes in blood velocity, which are presumed to directly measure changes in resistance of the artery (i.e., the lumen diameter change), occur nearly instantaneously in an event- related experimental paradigm, giving exceptional temporal resolution.

There remain several technical problems with fTDS. Only a limited number of large arteries can be imaged. Even in the arteries that are large enough and located within sight of the few available ultrasonic windows, the angle of the ultrasonic beam can make it very difficult to accurately measure blood flow changes. However, fTDS has several advantages over other functional neuro-imaging techniques including cost effectiveness; portability; continuous monitoring of blood flow activity; and excellent temporal resolution.

Functional Near-Infrared Spectroscopy

Functional near-infrared spectroscopy (fNIRS) is an emerging neuroimaging technology with several characteristics that make it a good candidate for use in military and intelligence applications. fNIRS uses light in the near infrared (700-900 nm), outside the visible spectrum, to measure changes in brain tissue that are associated with neuronal activity—in other words, it provides accurate spatial information about ongoing brain activity. Although fNIRS can measure several parameters associated with neural activity, the most common is the change in the ratio of oxygenated to deoxygenated hemoglobin in the blood, a measure analogous to fMRI's BOLD signal. Data from Huppert et al. (2006) demonstrate the relationship between the fMRI BOLD signal and fNIRS measures of deoxyhemoglobin (HbR), oxyhemoglobin (HbO), and total hemoglobin (HbT) (Figure 2-3). The design used a short-duration, event-related motor task, finger tapping, during the simultaneous recording of fMRI and fNIRS in five subjects. The results of Huppert et al. indicate that the fMRI-measured BOLD response is more highly correlated with the fNIRS measurement of deoxyhemoglobin than with the fNIRS measurement of oxyhemoglobin or total hemoglobin. This result was predicted from the theoretical basis of the BOLD response (as the BOLD response is based on changes in the concentration of HbR) and from previous publications (Toronov et al., 2001).

Using a more complex cognitive paradigm, target categorization, Bunce et al. (2006) replicated the fMRI protocol of McCarthy et al. (1997) using fNIRS. The results location and time course of McCarthy et al. are displayed in Figure 2-4, Row A. The fNIRS results were quite similar to the fMRI results reported by McCarthy et al. (1997).

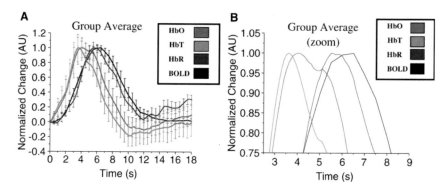

FIGURE 2-3 Averaged hemodynamic response function for simultaneously recorded fNIRS and BOLD responses during finger tapping. Maximum change was normalized to unity, and the HbR response was inverted. The error bars on plot (A) represent the standard error of each time point from the average. Plot (B) presents the first 8 sec of the same data to highlight the response peaks. The BOLD signal closely tracks the HbR measurement. SOURCE: Huppert et al. (2006). ©2006 by Elsevier. Reprinted with permission.

fNIRS has also been reported to measure changes in the optical properties of the cell membranes themselves that occur when a neuron fires (Gratton et al., 1995), referred to as an event-related optical signal (EROS). Although the signal-to-noise ratio is low in current technological incarnations, this latter measure is particularly interesting as it represents the holy grail of neuroimaging; high spatial resolution coupled to high temporal resolution. (Please see Appendix D for a more thorough discussion of fNIRS technology.)

Of importance in military applications, fNIRS is safe, noninvasive, and highly portable, even wireless. Subjects are able to sit upright, work on computers or perform other tasks, even walk on treadmills (Izzetoglu et al., 2004). With near-zero run-time costs, fNIRS is also inexpensive. Although current systems cost between $25,000 and $300,000, they are still largely bench-made. Continuous-wave systems could be manufactured for a few thousand dollars, and probably for less in volume, especially as the cost of manufacturing lasers and light-emitting diodes continues to fall (see Appendix D for further information on system types). Extant systems operate from a laptop computer and a 2 × 4 × 6 inch control box. Technological advances currently under development include having the entire system on a digital signal processing chip operating from a laptop computer and linked to a wireless sensor. These properties of fNIRS make neuroimaging possible where other neuroimaging technologies are impractical or impossible. Preliminary studies have been conducted with fNIRS in the backpacks of warfighters walking through virtual reality programs. Other advances currently under investigation include closed-loop human brain–computer interfaces and

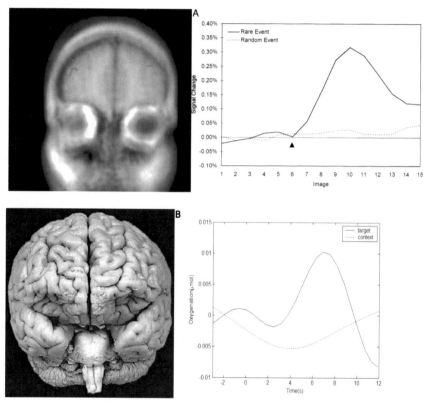

FIGURE 2-4 Replication of the fMRI protocol of McCarthy et al. (1997) using fNIRS. SOURCE: (A) McCarthy et al. (1997). ©1997 by the American Physiological Society; reprinted with permission. (B) (Image) Digital Anatomist images are from the Neuro-anatomy Interactive Syllabus, a project of the Structural Informatics Group, Department of Biological Structure, University of Washington, http://www9.biostr.washington.edu/da.html, by John W. Sundsten, Ph.D., and Kathleen A. Mulligan, Ph.D. Copyright 1998-2006 University of Washington, Seattle, Washington, U.S.A. All rights reserved including all photographs and images. No re-use, re-distribution, or commercial use without prior written permission of the authors and the University of Washington. (Graph) Bunce et al. (2006). ©2006 IEEE.

implantable optodes. Implantable optodes could allow realizing the holy grail of neuroimaging, the direct, noninvasive measurement of neuronal activity with millisecond-level time resolution and superior spatial resolution.

fNIRS measures relative changes in HbO and HbR, and total blood flow can be calculated from the differential equation. There are no approved clinical neuroimaging uses for this technique, but there are several advantages for experimental use. fNIRS systems are not as susceptible to movement artifact as fMRI, and algorithms are being refined for the removal of such artifacts (Izzetoglu et al., 2004). fNIRS depends on measurements of energy outside the visible spectrum. fNIRS was first used during World War I to monitor the blood oxygenation of bomber crews, a critical measurement before pressurized cabins were introduced in B-29s. Although fNIRS research has been ongoing since the late 1930s, the recent breakthroughs in both fNIRS and fMRI research have renewed interest in this technology. The capacity to translate findings from fMRI into fieldable, user-friendly, wearable devices is of significant interest. For instance, fNIRS has been shown to have promise in the detection of deception (Bunce et al., 2005), being both affordable and fieldable. The potential experimental uses of this technology are very exciting and include ecologically valid brain–computer interfaces; neurofeedback for guided facilitation of neural plasticity; and wearable neural monitors. Research groups in Japan (Haida et al., 2000), Ireland (Coyle et al., 2007), and the United States are working on brain–computer interfaces that allow locked-in patients (patients with no motor control, such as amyotrophic lateral sclerosis (ALS) patients) to communicate. In addition, Singapore has asked researchers in the United States to develop a brain fingerprint to identify specific brain signatures using fNIRS. Some advantages of the technology are its moderate cost (between \$25,000 and \$300,000) (Duscheck and Schandry, 2003) and its temporal resolution, which is similar to although somewhat lower than that of fMRI (1 cm^3).[13] It is also portable, wireless, and completely noninvasive.

These attributes allow fNIRS to be used with children and with patients who may find confinement in an fMRI magnet very unpleasant. A number of sensor applications exist, including caps, tension straps, and medical-grade adhesives. fNIRS is quiet and comfortable and therefore amenable to sensitive protocols such as the induction of positive moods and to integration with other technologies, including EEG. Appendix D provides additional information on the cost of the technology. NIRS can theoretically be combined with EEG, transcranial sonography, and other functional neuroimaging sensors. Unlike fMRI, where the subject is confined to the bore of the magnet, NIRS movement artifacts can be limited by proper affixation of sensors to the scalp. The major limitation is that NIRS best measures the first 2 or 3 centimeters of cortex so that deep brain imaging, at least through an intact skull, is challenging. Ongoing work, however, suggests that soon they will be able to image up to 5 cm deep.

Monitoring Advanced Cognitive Processes via Neuroimaging

There is a large body of published research on the use of various neuroimaging modalities to investigate the neural circuitry associated with deception.

---

[13]Currently, NIRs can localize hemodynamic changes within about 1 cm while the best fMRI scanner can localize changes within a few millimeters.

Recent PET and fMRI studies have provided insights, with specific areas in the prefrontal cortices and amygdala being the most commonly implicated regions (Abe et al., 2006, 2007; Mohamed et al., 2006; Davatzikos et al., 2005; Kozel et al., 2004a,b, 2005; Langleben et al., 2002, 2005; Lee et al., 2002, 2005; Nuñez et al., 2005; Phan et al., 2005a; Ganis et al., 2003; Spence et al., 2001). Recent NIRs studies of deception have also implicated prefrontal brain regions in the neural circuitry associated with deception (Bunce et al., 2005). Another recently published study that correlated fMRI measurements with standard skin conductance measurements during a concealed information paradigm had interesting results (Gamer et al., 2007). There are other possible uses for fMRI and other neuro-imaging technologies that would indirectly provide information about deception and that are far more likely to be successful in the near future. These indirect measures would not require any response from the subject but would provide passive information about the subject's experience. fMRI can already be used to judge recognition of items on a trial-by-trial basis. For example, one can imagine showing a subject a series of pictures of other people or crime scenes, and using fMRI to detect those that are familiar to the subject. The fMRI data could then be compared to the subject's own statements about familiarity; this would be an indirect measure of lying. Such trial-by-trial measures are already under active investigation in the fMRI field, and it is entirely possible that they could be enhanced to aid in detection of deception using targeted research funding.

Finding 2-5. Functional neuroimaging is progressing rapidly and is likely to produce important findings over the next two decades. For the intelligence community and the Department of Defense, two areas in which such progress could be of great interest are enhancing cognition and facilitating training. Additional research is still needed on states of emotion; motivation; psychopathology; language; imaging processing for measuring workload performance; and the differences between Western and non-Western cultures.

REFERENCES

Published

Abe, Nobuhito, Maki Suzuki, Etsuro Mori, Masatoshi Itoh, and Toshikatsu Fujii. 2007. Deceiving others: Distinct neural responses of the prefrontal cortex and amygdala in simple fabrication and deception with social interactions. *Journal of Cognitive Neuroscience* 19(2):287-295.
Abe, Nobuhito, Maki Suzuki, Takashi Tsukiura, Etsuro Mori, Keiichiro Yamaguchi, Masatoshi Itoh, and Toshikatsu Fujii. 2006. Dissociable roles of prefrontal and anterior cingulate cortices in deception. *Cerebral Cortex* 16(2):192-199.
Abraham, Michael H., Harpreet S. Chadha, and Robert C. Mitchell. 1994. Hydrogen bonding. 33. Factors that influence the distribution of solutes between blood and brain. *Journal of Pharmaceutical Sciences* 83(9):1257-1268.

Altoff, R.R., and Cohen, N.J. 1999. Eye-movement-based memory effect: Reprocessing effect in face perception. *Journal of Experimental Psychology: Learning, Memory and Cognition* 25: 997-1010.

Beduneau, A., P. Saulnier, N. Anton, F. Hindre, C. Passirani, H. Rajerison, N. Noiret, and J.P. Benoit. 2006. Pegylated nanocapsules produced by an organic solvent-free method: Evaluation of their stealth properties. *Pharmaceutical Research* 23(9):2190-2199.

Beecher, H.K. 1955. The powerful placebo. *Journal of the American Medical Association* 159:1602-1606.

Bentivoglio, Marina, and Krister Kristensson. 2007. Neural–immune interactions in disorders of sleep-wakefulness organization. *Trends in Neurosciences* 30(12):645-652.

Berger, H. 1929. Uber das elektrenkephalogramm des menschen. *Archiv fur Psychiatrie und Nervenkrankheiten* 87(1):527-580.

Blascovich, J. 2000. Psychophysiological methods. In *Handbook of Research Methods in Social and Personality Psychology*, H.T. Reis and C.M. Judd, eds. Cambridge, UK: Cambridge University Press.

Blascovich, J., and J. Tomaka. 1996. The biopsychosocial model of arousal regulation. In *Advances in Experimental Social Psychology*, M. Zanna, ed. New York, NY: Academic Press.

Blascovich, J., and M. Seery. 2007. Visceral and somatic indexes of social psychological constructs: History, principles, propositions, and case studies. In *Social Psychology: Handbook of Basic Principles*, A.W. Kruglanski and E.T. Higgins, eds. New York, NY: Guilford.

Born, Jan, Tanja Lange, Werner Kern, Gerard P. McGregor, Ulrich Bickel, and Horst L. Fehm. 2002. Sniffing neuropeptides: A transnasal approach to the human brain. *Nature Neuroscience* 5(6):514-516.

Bosi, Susanna, Tatiana Da Ros, Sabrina Castellano, Elena Banfi, and Maurizio Prato. 2000. Anti-mycobacterial activity of ionic fullerene derivatives. *Bioorganic and Medicinal Chemistry Letters* 10(10):1043-1045.

Brazier, Mary A.B. 1949. The electrical fields at the surface of the head during sleep. *Electroencephalography and Clinical Neurophysiology* 1(2; May):195-204.

Brightman, M.W., and T.S. Reese. 1969. Junctions between intimately apposed cell membranes in the vertebrate brain. *Journal of Cell Biology* 40(3):648-677.

Bunce, Scott C., Ajit Devaraj, Meltem Izzetoglu, Banu Onaral, and Kambiz Pourrezaei. 2005. Detecting deception in the brain: A functional near-infrared spectroscopy study of neural correlates of intentional deception. *Proceedings of SPIE* 5769:24-32.

Bunce, Scott C., Meltem Izzetoglu, Kurtulus Izzetoglu, Banu Onaral, and Kambiz Pourrezaei. 2006. Functional near-infrared spectroscopy: An emerging neuroimaging modality. *IEEE Engineering in Medicine and Biology Magazine* 25(4):54-62.

Cabeza, R., and L. Nyberg. 2000. Imaging cognition II: An empirical review of 275 PET and fMRI studies. *Journal of Cognitive Neuroscience* 12(1):1-47.

Cacioppo, J.T., and L.G. Tassinary. 1990a. *Principles of Psychophysiology: Physical, Social, and Inferential Elements*. New York: Cambridge University Press.

Cacioppo, J.T., and L.G. Tassinary. 1990b. Inferring psychological significance from physiological signals. *American Psychologist* 45(1):16-28.

Cacioppo, J.T., R.E. Petty, M.E. Losch, and H.S. Kim. 1986. Electromyographic activity over facial muscle regions can differentiate the valence and intensity of affective reactions. *Journal of Personality and Social Psychology* 50(2):260-268.

Cade, John F. 1949. Lithium salts in the treatment of psychotic excitement. *Medical Journal of Australia* 2:349-352.

Cao, Cong, Richard P. Suttmeier, and Denis Fred Simon. 2006. China's 15-year science and technology plan. *Physics Today* 59(12):38-43.

Carter, C. Sue. 1998. Neuroendocrine perspectives on social attachment and love. *Psychoneuroendocrinology* 23(8):779-818.

Carter, C. Sue, Margaret Altemus, and George P. Chrousos. 2001. Neuroendocrine and emotional changes in the post-partum period. *Progress in Brain Research* 133:241-249.

Chen, Robert J., Yuegang Zhang, Dunwei Wang, and Hongjie Dai. 2001. Noncovalent sidewall functionalization of single-walled carbon nanotubes for protein immobilization. *Journal of the American Chemical Society* 123(16):3838-3839.

Coyle, D., T.M. McGinnity, and G. Prasad. 2007. Identifying local ultrametricity of EEG time series for feature extraction in a brain-computer interface. Pp. 701-704 in *Proceedings of the 29th Annual International Conference of the IEEE Engineering in Medicine and Biology Society.*

Davatzikos, C., K. Ruparel, Y. Fan, D.G. Shen, M. Acharyya, J.W. Loughead, R.C. Gur, and D.D. Langleben. 2005. Classifying spatial patterns of brain activity with machine learning methods: Application to lie detection. *NeuroImage* 28(3):663-668.

Davis, P.A. 1939. Effects of acoustic stimuli on the waking human brain. *Journal of Neurophysiology* 2:494-499.

Dews, P.B., and G.R. Wenger. 1977. Rate-dependency of the behavioral effects of amphetamine. In *Advances in Behavioral Pharmacology*, Vol. 1, T. Thompson and P.B. Dews, eds. New York, NY: Academic Press.

Dickerson, B.C. 2007. Advances in functional magnetic resonance imaging: technology and clinical applications. *Neurotherapeutics* 4(3):360-70.

Dickerson, Sally S. and Margaret E. Kemeny. 2004. Acute stressors and cortisol responses: A theoretical integration and synthesis of laboratory research. *Psychological Bulletin* 130(3):355-391.

Dunning, Mark D., Andras Lakatos, Louiza Loizou, Mikko Kettunen, Charles French-Constant, Kevin M. Brindle, and Robin J.M. Franklin. 2004. Superparamagnetic iron oxide-labeled Schwann cells and olfactory ensheathing cells can be traced in vivo by magnetic resonance imaging and retain functional properties after transplantation into the CNS. *Journal of Neuroscience* 24(44):9799-9810.

Duscheck, Stephen, and Rainer Schandry. 2003. Functional transcranial Doppler sonography as a tool in psychophysiological research. *Psychophysiology* 40(3):436-54.

Ekman, Paul, and Maureen O'Sullivan. 2006. From flawed self-assessment to blatant whoppers: The utility of voluntary and involuntary behavior in detecting deception. *Behavioral Sciences and the Law* 24(5):673-686.

El Kaliouby, R., and P. Robinson. 2005. The Emotional Hearing Aid: An assistive tool for children with Asperger syndrome. *Universal Access in the Information Society* 4(2):121-134.

Ellis-Behnke, R.G., L.A. Teather, G.E. Schneider, and K.F. So. 2007. Using nanotechnology to design potential therapies for CNS regeneration. *Current Pharmaceutical Design* 13(24):2519-2528.

Emerich, Dwaine F., and Christopher G. Thanos. 2006. The pinpoint promise of nanoparticle-based drug delivery and molecular diagnosis. *Biomolecular Engineering* 23(4):171-184.

Estes, William. 2002. Traps in the route to models of memory and decision. *Psychonomic Bulletin and Review* 9(1):3-25.

Fender, D.H. 1987. Source localization of brain electrical activity. Pp. 355-403 in *Methods of Analysis of Brain Electrical and Magnetic Signals*, A.S. Gevins and A. Remond, eds. Amsterdam: Elsevier.

Feynman, Richard P. 1959. "There is plenty of room at the bottom," Lecture given at Annual Meeting of the American Physical Society, December 29, 1959, at California Institute of Technology, Pasadena, CA.

Floresco, Stan B., Mark A. Geyer, Lisa H. Gold, and Anthony A. Grace. 2005. Developing predictive animal models and establishing a preclinical trials network for assessing treatment effects on cognition in schizophrenia. *Schizophrenia Bulletin* 31(4):888-894.

Foer, Joshua. 2007. Remember this. *National Geographic* 212(5):32.

Fox, Daniel J., David F. Tharp, and Lydia C. Fox. 2005. Neurofeedback: An alternative and efficacious treatment for attention deficit hyperactivity disorder. *Applied Psychophysiology and Biofeedback* 30(4):365-373.

Frank, Mark G., and Paul Ekman. 2004. Appearing truthful generalizes across different deception situations. *Journal of Personality and Social Psychology* 86(3):486-495.

Freitas, Robert A., Jr. 1999. *Nanomedicine*, Vol. 1: *Basic Capabilities*. Austin, TX: Landes Bioscience.

Gamer, M., T. Bauermann, P. Stoeter, and G. Vossel. 2007. Covariations among fMRI, skin conductance, and behavioral data during processing of concealed information. *Human Brain Mapping* 28(12):1287-1301.

Ganis, G., S.M. Kosslyn, S. Stose, W.L. Thompson, and D.A. Yurgelun-Todd. 2003. Neural correlates of different types of deception: An fMRI investigation. *Cerebral Cortex* 13(8):830-836.

Gao, Xiaoling, Jun Chen, Weixing Tao, Jianhua Zhu, Qizhi Zhang, Hongzhuan Chen, and Xinguo Jiang. 2007a. UEA I-bearing nanoparticles for brain delivery following intranasal administration. *International Journal of Pharmaceutics* 340(1-2):207-215.

Gao, Xiaoling, Bingxian Wu, Qizhi Zhang, Jun Chen, Jianhua Zhu, Weiwei Zhang, Zhengxin Rong, Hongzhuan Chen, and Xinguo Jianga. 2007b. Brain delivery of vasoactive intestinal peptide enhanced with the nanoparticles conjugated with wheat germ agglutinin following intranasal administration. *Journal of Controlled Release* 121(3):156-167.

Golden, Pamela L., and Gary M. Pollack. 2003. Blood-brain barrier efflux transport. *Journal of Pharmaceutical Sciences* 92(9):1739-1753.

Goldstein, Alex S., John K. Amory, Stephanie M. Martin, Chris Vernon, Alvin Matsumoto, and Paul Yager. 2001. Testosterone delivery using glutamide-based complex high axial ratio microstructures. *Bioorganic and Medicinal Chemistry Letters* 9(11):2819-2825.

Gourley, Paul L. 2005. Brief overview of BioMicroNano technologies. *Biotechnology Progress* 21(1):2-10.

Grayson, Amy C.R., Insung S. Choi, Betty M. Tyler, Paul P. Wang, Henry Brem, Michael J. Cima, and Robert Langer. 2003. Multi-pulse drug delivery from a resorbable polymeric microchip device. *Nature Materials* 2(11):767-772.

Green, D.M., and J.A. Swets. 1966. *Signal Detection Theory and Psychophysics*. New York, NY: Wiley.

Guastella, Adam J., Phillip B. Mitchell, and Mark R. Dadds. 2008. Oxytocin increases gaze to the eye region of human faces. *Biological Psychiatry* 63(1):3-5.

Guertin, W.H., and P.L. Wilhelm. 1954. A statistical analysis of the electrodermal response employed in lie detection. *Journal of General Psychology* 51:153-160.

Gururangan, S., and H. Friedman. 2002. Innovations in design and delivery of chemotherapy for brain tumors. *Neuroimaging Clinics of North America* 12(4):583-597.

Hagan, J.J., and D.N. Jones. 2005. Predicting drug efficacy for cognitive deficits in schizophrenia. *Schizophrenia Bulletin* 31(4):830-853.

Haida, M., Y. Shinohara, Y. Ito, T. Yamamoto, F. Kawaguchi, and H. Koizumi. 2000. Brain function of an ALS patient in complete locked-in state by using optical topography. Pp. 95–97 in *The Frontier of Mind-Brain Science and Its Practical Applications (II)*, H. Koizumi, ed. Tokyo: Hitachi Ltd.

Hamaguchi, T., Y. Matsumura, M. Suzuki, K. Shimizu, R. Goda, I. Nakamura, I. Nakatomi, M. Yokoyama, K. Kataoka, and T. Kakizoe. 2005. NK105, a paclitaxel-incorporating micellar nanoparticle formulation, can extend in vivo antitumour activity and reduce the neurotoxicity of paclitaxel. *British Journal of Cancer* 92(7):1240-1246.

Hamilton, Alice. 1915. Lead poisoning in the manufacture of storage batteries. P. 27 in *Bulletin of the United States Bureau of Labor Statistics*, No. 165. Washington, D.C.: Government Printing Office.

Hammoud, D.A., J.M. Hoffman, and M.G. Pomper. 2007. Molecular neuroimaging: From conventional to emerging techniques. *Radiology* 245(1):21-42.

Heinrichs, Markus, Inga Neumann, and Ulrike Ehlert. 2002. Lactation and stress: Protective effects of breast-feeding in humans. *Stress* 5(3):195-203.

Heinrichs, Markus, Thomas Baumgartner, Clemens Kirschbaum, and Ulrike Ehlert. 2003. Social support and oxytocin interact to suppress cortisol and subjective responses to psychosocial stress. *Biological Psychiatry* 54(12):1389-1398.

Heinrichs, Markus, Gunther Meinlschmidt, Werner Wippich, Ulrike Ehlert, and Dirk H. Hellhammer. 2004. Selective amnesic effects of oxytocin on human memory. *Physiology and Behavior* 83(1):31-38.

Hillyer, Julián F., and Ralph M. Albrecht. 2001. Gastrointestinal persorption and tissue distribution of differently sized colloidal gold nanoparticles. *Journal of Pharmaceutical Sciences* 90(12):1927-1936.

Hirsch, Lee R., Naomi J. Halas, and Jennifer L. West. 2005. Whole-blood immunoassay facilitated by gold nanoshell-conjugate antibodies. *Methods in Molecular Biology* 303 (April):101-111.

Huber, Daniel, Pierre Veinante, and Ron Stoop. 2005. Vasopressin and oxytocin excite distinct neuronal populations in the central amygdala. *Science* 308(5719):245-248.

Huppert, T.J., R.D. Hoge, S.G. Diamond, M.A. Franceschini, and D.A. Boas. 2006. A temporal comparison of BOLD, ASL, and NIRS hemodynamic responses to motor stimuli in adult humans. *NeuroImage* 29(2):368-382.

Hussain, N., V. Jaitley, and A.T. Florence. 2001. Recent advances in the understanding of uptake of microparticulates across the gastrointestinal lymphatics. *Advanced Drug Delivery Reviews* 50(1):107-142.

Iacono, W.G. 2000. The detection of deception. *Handbook of Psychophysiology*, 2nd Ed., J.T. Cacioppo, L.G. Tassinary, and G.G. Berntson, eds. New York, NY: Cambridge University Press.

Illum, Lisbeth. 2000. Transport of drugs from the nasal cavity to the central nervous system. *European Journal of Pharmaceutical Sciences* 11(1):1-18.

Insel, Thomas R., and Larry J. Young. 2001. The neurobiology of attachment. *Nature Reviews Neuroscience* 2(2):129-136.

International Labour Office. 1934. Accumulators (storage batteries). P. 29 in *Occupation and Health: An Encyclopaedia of Hygiene, Pathology and Social Welfare*, Vol. 1. Geneva, Switzerland: International Labour Office.

Izzetoglu, K., S. Bunce, B. Onaral, K. Pourrezaei, and B. Chance. 2004. Functional optical brain imaging using NIR during cognitive tasks. *International Journal of Human-Computer Interaction* 17(2):211-227.

Jain, K.K. 2007. Nanobiotechnology-based drug delivery to the central nervous system. *Neurodegenerative Diseases* 4(4):287-291.

James, William. 1890. *Principles of Psychology*. Cambridge, MA: Harvard University Press.

Jarvik, Murray. 1970. Drugs used in the treatment of psychiatric disorders. *The Pharmacological Basis of Therapeutics*, L. Goodman and H. Gilman, eds. New York, NY: Macmillian.

Kleiman, M. 1992. *Against Excess: Drug Policy for Results*. New York, NY: Basic Books.

Koo, Yong-Eun E., Ramachandra G. Reddy, Mahaveer Bhojani, Randy Schneider, Martin A. Philbert, Alnawaz Rehemtulla, Brian D. Ross, and Raoul Kopelman. 2006. Brain cancer diagnosis and therapy with nanoplatforms. *Advanced Drug Delivery Reviews* 58(14):1556-1577.

Kosfeld, Michael, Markus Heinrichs, Paul J. Zak, Urs Fischbacher, and Ernst Fehr. 2005. Oxytocin increases trust in humans. *Nature* 435(7042):673-676.

Koushik, K., D.S. Dhanda, N.P.S. Cheruvu, and U.B. Kompella. 2004. Pulmonary delivery of deslorelin: Large-porous PLGA particles and HPbetaCD complexes. *Pharmaceutical Research* 21(7):1119-1126.

Kozak, Rouba, John P. Bruno, and Martin Sarter. 2006. Augmented prefrontal acetylcholine release during challenged attentional performance. *Cerebral Cortex* 16(1):9-17.

Kozel, F.A., T.M. Padgett, and M.S. George. 2004a. A replication study of the neural correlates of deception. *Behavioral Neuroscience* 118(4):852-856.

Kozel, F.A., Letty J. Revell, Jeffrey P. Lorberbaum, Ananda Shastri, Jon D. Elhai, Michael David Horner, Adam Smith, Ziad Nahas, Daryl E. Bohning, and Mark S. George. 2004b. A pilot study of functional magnetic resonance imaging brain correlates of deception in healthy young men. *Journal of Neuropsychiatry and Clinical Neurosciences* 16(3):295-305.

Kozel, F.A., K.A. Johnson, Q. Mu, E.L. Grenesko, S.J. Laken, and M.S. George. 2005. Detecting deception using functional magnetic resonance imaging. *Biological Psychiatry* 58(8):605-613.

Ladd, M.E. 2007. High-field-strength magnetic resonance: Potential and limits. *Topics in Magnetic Resonance Imaging* 18(2):139-152.

Landgraf, Rainer, and Inga D. Neumann. 2004. Vasopressin and oxytocin release within the brain: A dynamic concept of multiple and variable modes of neuropeptide communication. *Frontiers in Neuroendocrinology* 25(3-4):150-176.

Langleben, D.D., L. Schroeder, J.A. Maldjian, R.C. Gur, S. McDonald, J.D. Raglanda, C.P. O'Brien, and A.R. Childress. 2002. Brain activity during simulated deception: An event-related functional magnetic resonance study. *Neuroimage* 15(3):727-732.

Langleben, D.D., James W. Loughead, Warren B. Bilker, Kosha Rupare, Anna Rose Childress, Samantha I. Busch, and Ruben C. Gur. 2005. Telling truth from lie in individual subjects with fast event-related fMRI. *Human Brain Mapping* 26(4):262-272.

Langston, J. William. 1995. *The Case of the Frozen Addict.* New York, NY: Pantheon Press.

Lasagna L., F. Mosteller, J.M. von Felsinger, and H.K. Beecher. 1954. A study of the placebo response. *American Journal of Medicine* 16:770-779.

Lavie, N. 2005. Distracted and confused? Selective attention under load. *Trends in Cognitive Sciences* 9(2):75-82.

Lee, Tatia M.C., Ho-Ling Liu, Li-Hai Tan, Chetwyn C.H. Chan, Srikanth Mahankali, Ching-Mei Feng, Jinwen Hou, Peter T. Fox, and Jia-Hong Gao. 2002. Lie detection by functional magnetic resonance imaging. *Human Brain Mapping* 15(3):157-164.

Lee, Tatia M.C., Wen-hua Zhou, Xiao-jing Luo, Kenneth S.L. Yuen, Xin-zhong Ruan, and Xu-chu Weng. 2005. Neural activity associated with cognitive regulation in heroin users: A fMRI study. *Neuroscience Letters* 382(3):211-216.

Loo, C., L. Hirsch, M.H. Lee, E. Chang, J. West, N. Halas, and R. Drezek. 2005. Gold nanoshell bioconjugates for molecular imaging in living cells. *Optics Letters* 30(9):1012-1014.

Maloney, John M., Scott A. Uhland, Benjamin F. Polito, Norman F. Sheppard, Christina M. Pelta, and John T. Santini. 2005. Electrothermally activated microchips for implantable drug delivery and biosensing. *Journal of Controlled Release* 109(1-3):244-255.

Manji, H.K., J.M. Bebchuk, G.J. Moore, D. Glitz, K. Hasanat, G. Chen. 1999. Modulation of CNS signal transduction pathways and gene expression by mood stabilizing agents: Therapeutic implications. *Journal of Clinical Psychiatry* 60(S2):27-39.

Marchak, Frank M. 2006. Eye movement-based assessment of concealed knowledge. *Journal of Credibility Assessment and Witness Psychology* 7(2):148-163.

Martin, Charles R., and Punit Kohli. 2003. The emerging field of nanotube biotechnology. *Nature Reviews Drug Discovery* 2(1):29-37.

McCarthy, Gregory, Marie Luby, John Gore, and Patricia Goldman-Rakic. 1997. Infrequent events transiently activate human prefrontal and parietal cortex as measured by functional MRI. *Journal of Neurophysiology* 77(3):1630-1634.

Merkus, Frans W.H.M., and Mascha P. van den Berg. 2007. Can nasal drug delivery bypass the blood-brain barrier?: Questioning the direct transport theory. *Drugs in R & D* 8(3):133-144.

Michel, Christopher M., Micah M. Murray, Göran Lantz, Sara Gonzalez, Laurent Spinelli, and Rolando Grave de Peralta. 2004. EEG source imaging. *Clinical Neurophysiology* 115:2195-2222.

Miller, M.B., A. Kingstone, and M.S. Gazzaniga. 2002a. Hemispheric encoding asymmetries are more apparent than real. *Journal of Cognitive Neuroscience* 14(5):702-708.

Miller, M.B., J. Van Horn, G.L. Wolford, T.C. Handy, M. Valsangkar-Smyth, S. Inati, S. Grafton, and M.S. Gazzaniga. 2002b. Extensive individual differences in brain activations during episodic retrieval are reliable over time. *Journal of Cognitive Neuroscience* 14(8):1200-1214.

Miyata, N., and T. Yamakoshi. 1997. Fullerenes: Recent advances in the chemistry and physics of fullerenes and related materials. P. 345 in *Proceedings of the Symposium on Recent Advances in the Chemistry and Physics of Fullerenes and Related Materials*, Vol. 5, R.S. Ruoff and K.M. Kadish, eds. Pennington, NJ: Electrochemical Society.

Mohamed, Feroze B., Scott H. Faro, Nathan J. Gordon, Steven M. Platek, Harris Ahmad, and J. Michael Williams. 2006. Brain mapping of deception and truth telling about an ecologically valid situation: Functional MR imaging and polygraph investigation—initial experience. *Radiology* 238(2):679-688.

Moore, Gregory J. 1998. Proton magnetic resonance spectroscopy in pediatric neuroradiology. *Pediatric Radiology* 28(11):805-814.

Moore, Gregory J., J.M. Bebchuk, K. Hasanat, M.W. Faulk, N. Seraji-Bozorgzad, I.B. Wilds, C.L. Arfken, G. Chen, and H.K. Manji. 2000. Lithium increases N-acetyl-aspartate in the human brain: In vivo evidence in support of bcl-2's neurotrophic effects? *Biological Psychiatry* 48(1):1-8.

Musto, D. 1987. *The American Disease: Origins of Narcotic Control.* 2nd ed. New York, NY: Oxford University Press.

Nakada, T. 2007. Clinical application of high and ultra high-field MRI. *Brain and Development* 29(6):325-335.

Nishino, S. 2007a. Narcolepsy: Pathophysiology and pharmacology. *The Journal of Clinical Psychiatry* 68(Suppl. 13):9-15.

Nishino, S. 2007b. The hypocretin/orexin receptor: Therapeutic prospective in sleep disorders. *Expert Opinion on Investigational Drugs* 16(11):1785-1797.

Nitsche, Michael A., Christian Lampe, Andrea Antal, David Liebetanz, Nicolas Lang, Frithjof Tergau, and Walter Paulus. 2006. Dopaminergic modulation of long-lasting direct current-induced cortical excitability changes in the human motor cortex. *European Journal of Neuroscience* 23(6):1651-1657.

NRC (National Research Council). 2003. *The Polygraph and Lie Detection.* Washington, DC: The National Academies Press. Available from http://www.nap.edu/catalog.php?record_id=10420.

Nuñez, Jennifer Maria, B.J. Casey, Tobias Egner, Todd Hare, and Joy Hirsch. 2005. Intentional false responding shares neural substrates with response conflict and cognitive control. *NeuroImage* 25(1):267-277.

Olshansky, Brian. 2007. Placebo and nocebo in cardiovascular health. Implications for healthcare, research, and the doctor-patient relationship. *Journal of the American College of Cardiology* 49:415-421. Available from http://content.onlinejacc.org/cgi/reprint/49/4/415. Last accessed June 18, 2008.

OTA (Office of Technology Assessment of the U.S. Congress). 1983. *Scientific Validity of Polygraph Testing: A Research Review and Evaluation.* OTA-TM-H-15. Washington, DC: U.S. Congress.

OTA. 1990. *The Use of Integrity Tests for Pre-employment Screening.* OTA-SET-442. Washington, DC: U.S. Congress.

Panyam, Jayanth, and Vinod Labhasetwar. 2003. Biodegradable nanoparticles for drug and gene delivery to cells and tissue. *Advanced Drug Delivery Reviews* 55(3):329-347.

Pardridge, William M. 1999. Blood-brain barrier biology and methodology. *Journal of NeuroVirology* 5(6):556-569.

Pardridge, William M. 2001. BBB-genomics: Creating new openings for brain-drug targeting. *Drug Discovery Today* 6(8):381-383

Pedersen, Cort A. 1997. Oxytocin control of maternal behavior: Regulation by sex steroids and offspring stimuli. *Annals of the New York Academy of Sciences* 807:126-145.

Peters, David, Richard Genik, and Christopher Green. 2008. Neuroimaging in defense policy. Pp. 1-42 in *Biotechnology and the Future of America's Military: The "New" Biological Warfare*. Washington, DC: National Defense University Press.

Petrik, Vladimir, Vinothini Apok, Juliet Britton, B. Anthony Bell, and Marios Papadopoulos. 2006. Godfrey Hounsfield and the dawn of computed tomography. *Neurosurgery* 58(4):780-787.

Phan, K. Luan, Daniel A. Fitzgerald, Kunxiu Gao, Gregory J. Moore, Manuel E. Tancer, and Stefan Posse. 2004. Real-time fMRI of cortico-limbic brain activity during emotional processing. *NeuroReport* 15(3):527-532.

Phan, K. Luan, Alvaro Magalhaes, Timothy J. Ziemlewicz, Daniel A. Fitzgerald, Christopher Green, and Wilbur Smith. 2005a. Neural correlates of telling lies: A functional magnetic resonance imaging study at 4 tesla. *Academic Radiology* 12(2):164-172.

Phan, K. Luan, Daniel A. Fitzgerald, Pradeep J. Nathan, Gregory J. Moore, Thomas W. Uhde, and Manuel E. Tancer. 2005b. Neural substrates for voluntary suppression of negative affect: A functional magnetic resonance imaging study. *Biological Psychiatry* 57(3):210-219.

Phan, K. Luan, Daniel A. Fitzgerald, Bernadette M. Cortese, Navid Seraji-Bozorgzad, Manuel E Tancer, and Gregory J. Moore. 2005c. Anterior cingulate neurochemistry in social anxiety disorder: H-MRS at 4 tesla. *NeuroReport* 16(2):183-186.

Phelps, Michael E., Edward J. Hoffman, Nizar A. Mullani, and Michel M. Ter-Pogossian. 1975. Application of annihilation coincidence detection to transaxial reconstruction tomography. *Journal of Nuclear Medicine* 16(3):210-224.

Plonsey, R. 1963. Reciprocity applied to volume conductors and the ECG. *IEEE Transactions on Bio-Medical Engineering* 10(Jan.):9-12.

Poo, Mu-ming, and Aike Guo. 2007. Some recent advances in basic neuroscience research in China. *Philosophical Transactions of the Royal Society* 362:10.

Porges, Stephen W. 2006. The polygraph: One machine, two world views. *Journal of Credibility Assessment and Witness Psychology* 7:47-73.

Posse, Stefan, Daniel A. Fitzgerald, Kunxiu Gao, Ute Habel, David Rosenberg, Gregory J. Moore, and Frank Schneider. 2003. Real-time fMRI of temporolimbic regions detects amygdala activation during single-trial self-induced sadness. *NeuroImage* 18(3):760-768.

Prescott, James H., Sara Lipka, Samuel Baldwin, Norman F. Sheppard, John M. Maloney, Jonathan Coppeta, Barry Yomtov, Mark A. Staples, and John T. Santini. 2006. Chronic, programmed polypeptide delivery from an implanted, multireservoir microchip device. *Nature Biotechnology* 24(4):437-438.

Raichle, Marcus E. 2006. Neuroscience: The brain's dark energy. *Science* 314(5830):1249-1250.

Reese, T.S., and Morris J. Karnovsky. 1967. Fine structural localization of a blood-brain barrier to exogenous peroxidase. *Journal of Cell Biology* 34(1):207-217.

Robbins, T.W. 1998. Homology in behavioural pharmacology: An approach to animal models of human cognition. *Behavioural Pharmacology* 9:509-519.

Robbins, T.W. 2005. Chemistry of the mind: Neurochemical modulation of prefrontal cortical function. *Journal of Comparative Neurology* 493(1):140-146.

Rovner, Sophie L. 2007. Hold that thought. *Chemical and Engineering News* 85(36):13-20.

Sahankian, Barbara, and Sharon Morein-Zamir. 2007. Professor's little helper. *Nature* 450:1157-1159 and accompanying discussion. Available from http://www.nature.com/nature/journal/v450/n7173/full/4501157a.html. Last accessed 18 June 2008.

Santini, John T., Jr., Michael J. Cima, and Robert Langer. 1999. A controlled-release microchip. *Nature* 397(6717):335-338.

Sarter, M. 2006. Preclinical research into cognition enhancers. *Trends in Pharmacological Sciences* 27(11):602-608.

Sarter, M., and J Bruno. 1994. Cognitive functions of cortical ACh: Lessons from studies on trans-synaptic modulation of activated efflux. *Trends in Neurosciences* 17(6):217-221.

Saul, Stephanie. 2007. Sleep drugs found only mildly effective, but wildly popular. *The New York Times,* October 23, 2007.

Shapiro, D., and A. Crider. 1969. Psychophysiological approaches in social psychology. In *Handbook of Social Psychology,* Vol. III. (2nd Edition), G. Lindzey and E. Aronson, eds. Reading, MA: Addison-Wesley.

Shaw, J.C., and M. Roth. 1955. Potential distribution analysis. I. A new technique for the analysis of electrophysiological phenomena. *Electroencephalography and Clinical Neurophysiology* 7(2; May):273-284.

Silva, Gabriel A. 2006. Neuroscience nanotechnology: Progress, opportunities and challenges. *Nature Reviews Neuroscience* 7(1):65-74.

Silva, Gabriel A. 2007. Nanotechnology approaches for drug and small molecule delivery across the blood brain barrier. *Surgical Neurology* 67(2):113-116.

Society for Neuroscience. 2007. *Annual Meeting Statistics*. Society for Neuroscience 2007. Available from http://www.sfn.org/index.cfm?pagename=annualMeeting_statistics&section=annualMeeting. Last accessed June 18, 2008.

Spence, S.A., T.F. Farrow, A.E. Herford, I.D. Wilkinson, Y. Zheng, and, P.W. Woodruff. 2001. Behavioural and functional anatomical correlates of deception in humans. *NeuroReport* 12(13):2849-2853.

Spence, S.A., M.D. Hunter, T.F. Farrow, R.D. Green, D.H. Leung, C.J. Hughes, and V. Ganesan. 2004. A cognitive neurobiological account of deception: Evidence from functional neuroimaging. *Philosophical Transactions of the Royal Society of London, Series B, Biological Sciences* 359(1451):1755-1762.

Strand, Fleur L. 1999. *Neuropeptides: Regulators of Physiological Processes*. Cambridge, MA: MIT Press.

Suri, Sarabjeet Singh, Hicham Fenniri, and Baljit Singh. 2007. Nanotechnology-based drug delivery systems. *Journal of Occupational Medicine and Toxicology* 2:16.

Swazey, Judith P. 1974. *Chlorpromazine in Psychiatry: A Study of Therapeutic Innovation*. Cambridge, MA: MIT Press.

Tabata, Yasuhiko, Yoshiyuki Murakami, and Yoshito Ikada. 1997a. Photodynamic effect of polyethylene glycol-modified fullerene on tumor. *Japanese Journal of Cancer Research* 88(11):1108-1116.

Tabata, Yasuhiko, Yoshiyuki Murakami, and Yoshito Ikada. 1997b. Antitumor effect of poly(ethylene glycol)-modified fullerene. *Fullerenes, Nanotubes and Carbon Nanostructures* 5(5):989-1007.

Taleb, Nassim Nicholas. 2007a. *The Black Swan: The Impact of the Highly Improbable*. New York, NY: Random House.

Teixido, Meritxell, and Ernest Giralt. 2008. The role of peptides in blood-brain barrier nanotechnology. *Journal of Peptide Science* 14(2):163-173.

Ter-Pogossian, M.M, M.E. Phelps, and E.J. Hoffman. 1975. A positron-emission transaxial tomograph for nuclear imaging (PETT). *Radiology* 114(1):89-98.

Torche, A.M., H. Jouan, P. Le Corre, E. Albina, R. Primault, A. Jestin, and R. Le Verge. 2000. Ex vivo and in situ PLGA microspheres uptake by pig ileal Peyer's patch segment. *International Journal of Pharmaceutics* 201(1):15-27.

Toronov, V.A.W., J.H. Choi, M. Wolf, A. Michalos, E. Gratton, and D. Hueber. 2001. Investigation of human brain hemodynamics by simultaneous near-infrared spectroscopy and functional magnetic resonance imaging. *Medical Physics* 28(4):521-527.

Tsao, Nina, Puthuparampil P. Kanakamma, Tien-Yau Luh, Chen-Kung Chou, and Huan-Yao Lei. 1999. Inhibition of *Escherichia coli*-induced meningitis by carboxyfullerene. *Antimicrobial Agents and Chemotherapy* 43(9):2273-2277.

Tsao, Nina, Tien-Yau Luh, Chen-Kung Chou, Jiunn-Jong Wu, Yee-Shin Lin, and Huan-Yao Lei. 2001. Inhibition of group A streptococcus infection by carboxyfullerene. *Antimicrobial Agents and Chemotherapy* 45(6):1788-1793.

Tsiamyrtzis P., J. Dowdall, D. Shastri, I.T. Pavlidis, M.G. Frank, and P. Ekman. 2007. Imaging facial physiology for the detection of deceit. *International Journal of Computer Vision* 71(2): 197-214.

Uvnäs-Moberg, Kerstin. 1998. Oxytocin may mediate the benefits of positive social interaction and emotions. *Psychoneuroendocrinology* 23(8):819-835.

Van Der Lubben, I.M., F.A. Konings, G. Borchard, J.C. Verhoef, and H.E. Junginger. 2001. In vivo uptake of chitosan microparticles by murine Peyer's patches: Visualization studies using confocal laser scanning microscopy and immunohistochemistry. *Journal of Drug Targeting* 9(1):39-47.

Varde, Neelesh K., and Daniel W. Pack. 2004. Microspheres for controlled release drug delivery. *Expert Opinion on Biological Therapy* 4(1):35-51.

Weissleder, Ralph, Kimberly Kelly, Eric Yi Sun, Timur Shtatland, and Lee Josephson. 2005. Cell-specific targeting of nanoparticles by multivalent attachment of small molecules. *Nature Biotechnology* 23(11):1418-1423.

White, Barbara Prudhomme, Kathryn A. Becker-Blease, and Kathleen Grace-Bishop. 2006. Stimulant medication use, misuse, and abuse in an undergraduate and graduate student sample. *Journal of American College Health* 54(5):261-268.

Wilson, Edward O. 1998. *Consilience: The Unity of Knowledge*. New York, NY: Knopf Publishing Group.

Young, Larry J., Miranda M. Lim, Brenden Gingrich, and Thomas R. Insel. 2001. Cellular mechanisms of social attachment. *Hormones and Behavior* 40(2):133-138.

Zak, Paul J., and Ahlam Fakhar. 2006. Neuroactive hormones and interpersonal trust: International evidence. *Economics and Human Biology* 4(3):412-429.

Zak, Paul J., Angela A. Stanton, and Sheila Ahmadi. 2007. Oxytocin increases generosity in humans. *PLoS ONE* 2(11):e1128.

Unpublished

Barrett, James. "Trends and Developments in Neuropsychopharmacology: A 20-year Perspective." Presentation to the committee on August 15, 2007.

Chatterjee, Anjan. "Cosmetic Neurology." Presentation to the committee on August 15, 2007.

Dinges, David. "Optimizing Neurobehavioral Performance though Biology and Technology." Presentation to the committee on August 15, 2007.

Imrey, Peter. "Signal Detection Theory: How Bayes' Theorem Constrains Accuracy of Inference from Neurophysiologic Monitoring." Presentation to the committee on October 31, 2007.

Kelly, Tom. "Experimental Methods in Clinical Neuropsychopharmacology." Presentation to the committee on August 15, 2007.

Miller, Mike. "Unique Patterns of Individual Brain Activity." Presentation to the committee on October 31, 2007.

Raichle, Marcus. 2007. "Two Views of Brain Function." Presentation to the committee on October 31, 2007.

Simon, Denis. 2007. "Scientific Innovation and Investment in China." Presentation to the committee on August 15, 2007.

Taleb, Nassim Nicholas. 2007b. Nassim Nicholas Taleb's home page 2007 [cited December 13, 2007]. Available from http://www.fooledbyrandomness.com/. Last accessed on June 18, 2008.

3

Emerging Areas of Cognitive Neuroscience and Neurotechnologies

INTRODUCTION

Much of the foundation of current neuroscience research is discussed in Chapter 2. In Chapter 3, the discussion is expanded to include potential applications for neuroscience that may emerge in the next two decades. The committee points out that the two areas it covers in this chapter—computational biology and distributed human-machine systems—are not meant to represent the entire spectrum of possibilities. Rather, they are areas the committee selected as examples. Some of these applications are already beginning to appear and may one day impact the intelligence and military communities.

COMPUTATIONAL BIOLOGY APPLIED TO COGNITION, FUNCTIONAL NEUROIMAGING, GENOMICS, AND PROTEOMICS

While computing is essentially ubiquitous in the fields of neuroscience and cognition, it can broadly be said to have impact in two areas. The first is analysis, with computation used to analyze the enormous quantities of data acquired from genome sequencing, neuroimaging, ribonucleic acid (RNA) expression arrays, and the study of proteomics, and to correlate them with experimental conditions to eventually understand the biology of the nervous system and cognition. Analysis broadly includes what falls traditionally in the areas of bioinformatics.

The second area where computation has an impact is modeling. It entails putting a hypothesis into concrete computational form in an attempt to validate the hypothesis and/or make a prediction. In biophysical models the physical behavior of the system is modeled, and in biomathematical models the quantities associated with the system are abstracted mathematically and studied. In some cases, a model is of both kinds. The distinction between the two kinds of models is not always sharp because data analysis often/sometimes makes basic assumptions about the data fitting a specific model. To understand how the two categories are affected by the limitations of computational technology, each is first discussed separately. Then the concerns that are apparent when they are considered together are discussed.

Analysis of Experimental Data

The analysis of genetic data,[1] proteome data,[2] morphologic data,[3] and neuro-imaging data[4] is the most common use of computation in neuroscience. Computing has played a critical role in enabling the technologies that produce these data. This role ranges from data acquisition to creating the algorithms used to tease the signals out of the data.

The hardware requirements for analyzing large data sets are relatively straightforward. Applications based on database search and local alignment depend on a style of high-performance computing (HPC) known as "embarrassingly parallel."[5] This generally requires between 10 and 1,000 identical servers, each of which is given a portion of the search and alignment task to accomplish. Embarrassingly parallel computing requires little coordination between servers. The cost of HPC clusters is now well within the reach of individual departments and research groups owing to the emergence of Beowulf-class computer clusters, which are built on commodity hardware deploying Linux operating systems and open source software.[6]

The challenges lie in the development of software programs for analysis of large data sets. This requires advances in the science of bioinformatics, also known as computational biology. Bioinformatics is a multidisciplinary field at the intersection of computer science, statistics and molecular biology. Neuroscience

---

[1] Sources of genetic data are microarrays, whole genome sequences, and epigenetic changes, among others.

[2] An example of proteome data is data that comes from mass spectroscopy.

[3] Morphologic data comes from quantitation of cells, phenotyping, and locating over time.

[4] Techniques that generate functional neuroimaging data include electroencephalography (EEG), magnetoencephalography (MEG), functional magnetic resonance imaging (fMRI), positron emission tomography (PET), and near-infrared spectroscopy (NIRs).

[5] "Embarrassingly parallel" tasks typically include doing an identical problem over and over again with different starting configurations or different random seeds. In these cases, there is generally little or no communication between the different processors. For additional information, see the Web site of the University of Melbourne's Department of Computer Science and Software Engineering at http://www.cs.mu.oz.au/498/notes/node40.html. Last accessed on January 18, 2008.

[6] "Beowulf clusters" describes a set of identical computing nodes that are connected together somewhat loosely in order to enable communication between the nodes. In general, the individual nodes are off-the-shelf computers connected to one another through a commodity means (usually just Ethernet). For additional information, see the Beowulf Project Overview Web site at http://www.beowulf.org/overview/index.html. Last accessed on January 18, 2008.

benefits from the developments of analytical techniques that are applicable to data from many areas of biology, such as genomics and proteomics. The science has evolved to allow the large-scale integration of data from a variety of sources for analysis of complete complex systems rather than individual parts (Drabløs et al., 2004).[7] For instance, algorithms have been developed to assemble and align genome sequences, to identify genes and their functions, to analyze data from large-scale expression arrays, and to build integrated databases.[8]

There should be a significant role for computing in the analysis of neuro-imaging data. It is somewhat remarkable that computing has not played a larger role in neuroimaging data analysis. In many ways, the field should be one of the most important scientific drivers for high-performance computing. Imaging data sets are among the largest sets of data produced by any scientific field. Additionally, distinguishing the signals from the noise is extremely complicated in neuroimaging data. However, neuroimaging analysis has been somewhat reluctant compared to other kinds of computations analysis to apply state-of-the-art scientific computing techniques. Significant breakthroughs might occur if massively parallel computing were applied to analyzing the neuroimaging data that currently exist, but there is still no significant effort to engage computational resources at such a scale to solve this problem. The mathematical effort that is being applied in the area is somewhat closer to the state of the art in that field, but again, a push by the neuroimaging community to engage more applied mathematicians could well lead to improved results.

There is a fundamental limitation, however, on the potential for breakthroughs in neuroimaging analysis. It is impossible to detect the electrical or magnetic signals at a certain temporal and spatial resolution given the shielding provided by the skull and brain. In the case of magnetic imaging, the fields that are used to stimulate natural magnetic activity in the brain are already thought to be close to the limit of human safety. Although one might surmise that advances in magnet technology could lead to much higher resolution, it would probably be too dangerous to perform these experiments on human subjects. As long as these temporal and spatial resolutions lie above those needed for individual neuronal monitoring, interpreting the experimental data will have to rely on assumptions. There is potential for improved electrodes that could be inserted directly into the brain to do very precise monitoring of individual neurons, but it is extremely unlikely that such technology could be used for anything other than very small doses without significantly damaging the subject. For this reason one would have

---

[7]For additional information, see Drabløs et al. (2004) at http://www.ime.ntnu.no/infosam2020/ oldpage/work_groups/wg_bioinformatics.html). Last accessed on January 4, 2008.

[8]A completely inclusive list would also include protein modifications, protein-protein/protein-nucleic/and protein-lipid interactions, gene regulation through alternative splicing and microRNAs, and multi-scalar integration to deduce and predict signaling pathways and information networks; however, given the fact that new technologies are being developed constantly, the committee chose to limit this list to a few of the most widely used key technologies as representative examples.

to be extremely cautious about predicting revolutionary improvements in gathering neuroscience data in the next two decades.

Physiologically Plausible Models of Human Cognition and Affect

Modeling and simulation represent an entirely different way to apply computation to cognitive and neural sciences, and here the future is much harder to predict. While data analysis will most likely be limited in the near term by the physical limitations associated with data collection, modeling will in some respects be limited only by the resources that any group would choose to devote to it.

Building a neurophysiologically plausible model of the whole brain will most likely remain impossible for the near future. Because it is now possible to model large neuronal networks with biophysically detailed neurons and synaptic properties that approach the numbers and complexity found in living nervous systems (Silver et al., 2007), it is tempting to predict computational power in 20 years based with the typical number of neurons in a human brain. This would be a deceptive comparison, however, for the primary difficulty in building a model of the brain is not the lack of computational power but inadequate understanding of how to model in detail the neurophysiological, cognitive, and affective aspects of brain function. Despite tremendous advances in general understanding of how individual parts of the brain work and communicate among themselves, it is highly unlikely under current assumptions that research breakthroughs allowing a neurophysiologically plausible model of a whole brain will occur in the next two decades. This is not just because the relationship among parts of the brain is so complex, but is also because collective understanding of the relationship between the observed neurophysiological aspects of the brain and the more subtle questions associated with human cognition is so limited. Moreover, the brain is not a standalone organ but interacts in complex ways with monitoring and regulatory systems throughout the body. The committee does not wish to imply that a fairly comprehensive understanding of the neural systems (including the brain) of other simpler organisms will not be gained in the next two decades. It is not unreasonable to believe that a simple model organism such as *C. elegans* will have its neural system understood in two decades, or that studies on transgenic animals such as mice will not yield additional understanding about mammalian brains in general. However, given the, in many ways, unique nature of the human neural system and the difficulty of doing experiments with similar or equivalent organisms, even the best such work would still not yield data on important aspects of the human neural system.

Based on its current understanding, the committee hopes and expects that neuroimaging technology will eventually demonstrate a relatively straightforward neural architecture that can be implemented in a computational model, but such an imaging technology will most likely require a spatial and temporal resolution well beyond anything that currently exists or will exist in the near future. Of course, it is also very possible that the architecture of the brain could turn out to be something that is very difficult to simulate using today's digital or analog computing architectures.

High-fidelity modeling of the human brain will require breakthroughs in collective understanding of how to model cognition and affect. Approaches to this challenge are likely to leverage the property of emergence, which is found in many natural systems—that is, the ability of these systems to generate adaptive complexity by means of elegant simpler principles. The principle of emergent behavior is especially complex with respect to future predictions. It is likely to play a key role in the ultimate understanding of how the brain works, but no one has been able to capture it in a way that fits current understanding of brain function. But given emergent behavior's importance, it is very important to recognize that organizations and nations that are able to harness their creativity, expertise in cognitive neurosciences, and computational resources to such an end will have a large degree of leverage in defining the next revolution in technology (Goldstein, 1999).

Finding 3-1. The global scientific computing community is approaching an era in which high-end computing will, in principle, be sufficient in capacity and computational power to model the human brain. However, there does not yet exist either an adequate and detailed understanding of *how* such modeling can be done, or a complete model of how the brain interacts with complex regulatory and monitoring systems throughout the body. These and other difficulties make it highly unlikely that in the next two decades anyone could build a neurophysiologically plausible model of the whole brain and its array of specialized and general-purpose higher cognitive functions.

Proteomics and Genomics

Science of Genomics and Proteomics

There are additional computational methodologies that will drive fundamental understanding of how the brain works. They will be concentrated in genomics and proteomics. Any discussion of modern biology must refer to the revolutionary role that genomics and proteomics are playing, and will continue to play, over the next few decades.

Neuroscience, and biology in general, has until recently been considered to be an observational science. The fundamental paradigm was making observations of a system or parts of it and correlating those observations with a specific behavior or result. Qualitative rules were then developed that could be applied with some fidelity to draw conclusions about what role each part of the system played in the whole system. One could also begin to describe how variations in

each of these parts drove differences between different organisms within a specific species and how one species differed from another. This approach, carried
on in a heroic way during the nineteenth and twentieth centuries by outstanding
biologists, led to a remarkable knowledge base for many different aspects of
biological science. However, it was very difficult to use these broad observations
to build a formal set of rules that could be used to gain a greater understanding
of the system as a whole. Perhaps even more important, this work did not give
significant insight into the mechanisms that determined *why* these variations
appeared from organism to organism.

The genomics revolution has changed this picture remarkably. While the fundamental role of genes has been understood since the time of Mendel, the ability
by scientists to decode individual genomes letter for letter has become a powerful
tool for biology and neuroscience. [9] It allows one to build a quantitative scientific
basis for understanding the effect of specific, well-defined, and easily measured
genomic sequences on traits or behavior. Furthermore, it allows what is known
as comparative genomics, which is the science of understanding relationships
between genomes of different species or strains within a species. This powerful
tool is not useful just for its ability to classify differences, but it allows experiments to be done on one species that can be somewhat faithfully extrapolated to
other species. Because of the simple four-letter alphabet of genomics, computers
can be used to make quantitative predictions about the behavior and traits of
individuals based just on their genome. This is a tremendous improvement over
a system of more qualitative observations.

More importantly, genomics is enabling not only an understanding of what
determines differences from organism to organism but also a mechanistic understanding of why the individual differences occur and what the mechanism is that
causes the differences. It is a tenet of biology that the expression of genes occurs
to a large extent through their manifestation as the instruction code for building
the proteins that make up the fundamental machinery of cells. Gene expression
can be analyzed at the single cell level to provide insights into how neurons and
glial cells respond to different physiologic signals and also to characterize regional
differences in the same types of cells (Ng et al., 2007). High-throughput methods
permit genome-wide searches to discover genes that are uniquely expressed in
brain circuits and regions that control behavior in animal model systems. In situ
hybridization then permits anatomic localization of the expressed genes. [10]

However, not all genes that are expressed are translated into proteins. The
study of proteins is known as proteomics, and it provides an even closer link

---

[9]Gregor Mendel, a 19th century plant geneticist, discovered the underlying principles of heredity
common to all life forms. While understanding the fundamental role that genes play was the result
of work of the greater scientific community that occurred largely after Mendel, his initial work was
seminal.

[10]For additional information, see the Allen Brain Atlas of the Allen Institute for Brain Science's at
http://www.brain-map.org. Last accessed on January 4, 2008.

to the understanding of the fundamental physical basis for processes in cells. The computational questions surrounding proteomics are generally even more complex than those of genomics and focus on developing complex graphs of protein interactions representing metabolic function. Because a protein's structure determines its function, there are also additional computational needs related to graphing a protein structure at the molecular level to better understand the function it performs.

Implications of Proteomics and Genomics Research for Neuroscience

Probably the most obvious and talked about impact that genomics research will have on neuroscience is in the area of genetic testing. Once significant genomic information is available about the general human population, as there will be in 20 years time, correlating genetic markers not only with intelligence but also with the ability to learn and be trained to perform a variety of specific physical and mental tasks will become a relatively straightforward exercise.[11] Such screening would allow the objective identification of the differential vulnerability of people to intense stress, sleep loss, drug effects, hypoxia, and dehydration. It would be a tremendous advantage to any organization to start with a pool of trainees who had been selected via genetic screening such that most of them, not just 1 to 10 percent, would go on to perform a given task in an outstanding manner. The abilities could include such things as learning a foreign language, performing a task on limited amounts of sleep, and performing as an elite athlete. Currently, screening for such abilities is done through different types of testing, but to a large extent they measure the existing aptitude, not the inherent potential.

It is important to point out that while the potential for genetic screening exists, there is no guarantee that a gene or genes exist that will directly control the trait of interest. It is widely understood, for instance that "intelligence" is a difficult characteristic to define, and it is unlikely that a small set of genes would be an indicator of intelligence. It may even turn out that, for all traits of interest, the effect of the genes is negligible compared to the effect of the environment. Of even greater concern would be the incorrect use of genetic testing so that excellent candidates are turned away due to a badly validated testing procedure.

Proteomics provides an extremely strong scientific framework for understanding the effect of neuroenhancing pharmaceuticals. As the designing of

---

[11]The key point is that doing the correlation itself will be a relatively straightforward exercise. The result of the exercise will often be that the correlation is weak to non-existent. It is important to emphasize that strong correlations will not necessarily be found, but that it will be easy to do such a search and, if such correlations exist, they will be easy to find. The committee does not doubt that there will probably be disappointment in those who are looking for simple genetic correlations with broad traits. At the same time, the committee would not be surprised if there were a few remarkable correlations found with a handful of traits.

drugs becomes more computational and less a matter of hit-and-miss testing, understanding the structure and function of the proteins of interest in the relevant pathways becomes a vital piece of the drug design puzzle. One can begin to rationally design active molecules based on the structure of the molecular actors of interest. Additionally, one can understand the effect on the larger metabolic system of shutting down a particular pathway so that side effects can be better understood from the start. As the metabolic machinery of the brain becomes better understood and metabolic engineering and proteomics become understood jointly in a systems fashion, it is possible that neuroenhancing (or perhaps even neurodefensive) compounds could make a significant leap forward. It is important to note, however, that rational drug design is and most likely will remain a very difficult endeavor.

Genomics and proteomics are already making certain aspects of imaging significantly easier. One aspect of this is the creation of transgenic mice, which have been engineered to express different fluorescent proteins in different situations. This allows the visualization of specific cellular behaviors in live animals under realistic conditions. Such research holds tremendous value for the real-time imaging of neural activity in animals that could in turn be used to understand similar neural activity in people. It also serves as evidence of the power and potential of genetic engineering. It should be noted that the techniques involved in adding fluorescent markers to proteins are much better understood than the general genetic enhancement which has been speculated about in the literature. It is not out of the question, however, that advances in genomics could enable more significant advances in genetic engineering. Current ethical constraints, combined with the significantly longer life-cycle of humans, make it unlikely that such work have an effect in the next two decades. Finally, as knowledge of these subjects grows, it may be possible to predict much more about individual abilities, capabilities, personality characteristics, and other traits from the genome; such information may be particularly useful to the intelligence community and the military.[12]

DISTRIBUTED HUMAN-MACHINE SYSTEMS

Advances in neurophysiological and cognitive science research have fueled a surge of research aimed at more effectively combining human and machine capabilities. Results of this research could give human performance an edge at both the individual and group levels. Though much of this research defies being assigned rigid boundaries between disciplines, for the sake of convenience the committee has organized this section into four discussion areas:

---

[12]There is no doubt in the mind of the committee members that genomics and proteomics will play an increasingly large role in the future of cognitive neuroscience. However, given the fact that genomics/proteomics is largely recognized by the entire technical community as being important, and appears to be growing, the committee decided to not add a finding related to this topic.

• *Brain-machine interfaces*. This category includes direct brain-machine interfaces for control of hardware and software systems. Traditional human interface technologies, such as visualization (Thomas and Cook, 2005), are not considered in this report.

• *Robotic prostheses and orthotics*. Included here are replacement body parts (robotic prostheses) and mechanical enhancement devices (robotic orthotics) designed to improve or extend human performance in the physical domain.

• *Cognitive and sensory prostheses*. These technologies are designed to improve or extend human performance in the cognitive domain through sensory substitution and enhancement capabilities or by continually sensing operator state and providing transparent augmentation of operator capabilities.

• *Software and robotic assistants*. These technologies also are designed to improve or extend human performance in the physical and/or cognitive domains. However, unlike the first three areas for discussion, they achieve their effect by interacting with the operator(s) rather than as assistants or team members in the manner of a direct prosthetic or orthotic extension of the human body, brain, or senses. Agent-based technologies for social and psychological simulations are not considered in this report.

Brain-Machine Interfaces

The basis of brain-machine interfaces (BMI) is the capture of various forms of dynamically varying energy emissions from the working brain by means of functional neuroimaging devices. These devices include the electroencephalograph (EEG) and the magnetoencephalograph (MEG) for the detection of the electrical energy of working neurons; functional near-infrared spectroscopy (fNIRS), which uses light to measure the hemodynamic response of functional regions of the brain, and functional magnetic resonance imaging (fMRI), which uses powerful magnetic fields to detect magnetic resonance differences in blood in different areas of the brain and allows them to be correlated to differences in neuronal activity (i.e., oxygen consumption). Positron emission tomography (PET) uses a gamma ray detector that locates and records bioactive radioactive assays injected into the blood, thereby measuring the metabolism of neurons in the functional regions of the brain.

The brain is so remarkably flexible that people can, after just a few hours of feedback training, learn to activate and deactivate functional regions and to vary the brain's electrical distribution, metabolic activity, and brain wave patterns. A BMI takes advantage of neuroplasticity to activate and control electronic or mechanical devices (Birbaumer, 2006). A surprising amount of work is being done on connecting the brain directly to prosthetics. EEG and MEG scanners can record oscillation signals from the whole brain or functionally specific regions and activate a device when the subject specifically controls this activity. Slow cortical potentials (SCPs) and sensorimotor rhythm (SMR) have both been used to activate electronic devices. Evoked potentials recorded by EEG, especially the positive deflecting waveform that occurs approximately 300 msec following an evoked potential (P300 wave), have been used to activate and even operate communications equipment (Birbaumer, 2007). The blood-oxygenation-level-dependent (BOLD) magnetic resonance (MR) signal and NIRs instruments measuring cortical blood flow have also been used as a BMI (Birbaumer, 2007). Reinforcement learning and other algorithmic techniques have been used to rapidly identify the neural signatures of intentional actions and train BMI machine learning subsystems (DiGiovanna et al., 2007). Much of the research to date has had the objective of enabling people to exert some degree of control over a prosthetic, pointing, or communication device (Schwartz, 2004).

Neuroplasticity is the critical basis for this work. The working brain adapts its functioning very quickly and readily given adequate, timely, and veridical feedback even with informal training. With operant conditioning the brain can quickly learn and adapt to new kinds of interaction demands (Bach-y-Rita, 1996). However, the limits of neuroplasticity are still poorly misunderstood.

Another important issue is the complexity of response that can be driven by BMIs. While it is beyond the scope of this report to attempt to quantify the relative complexity of using a human hand and arm to the high-level operation of an aircraft, the committee speculates that given sufficiently rich sensorimotor feedback (essentially a sensory prosthetic—see below), the levels of complexity may be within the same order of magnitude. However, the training and detection-of-brain-activity capabilties needed to bring BMIs to this level of complexity and specificity are still beyond current technical reach, and the ultimate range of the associated physiological potential and limitations is not yet well understood. More important, from the point of view of enhancement (vs. rehabilitation) of human performance, it has not yet been established that BMI is superior to other methods of direct control of computing functions and robotic vehicles. Promising areas for continued BMI research include the control of robotic orthotics (see section "Robotic Prosthetics and Orthotics") and the management of information flow to an individual based on changes in the user's cognitive state (see the section "Cognitive Prostheses").

Finding 3-2. Research on brain-machine interfaces (BMIs) has progressed steadily, with the principal objective being to allow people to exert some degree of control over a prosthetic, pointing and tracking, or communication device. The ultimate range of physiological potential and limitations for BMIs is not yet well understood. From the point of view of enhancement (versus rehabilitation) of human performance, it has not yet been established that BMI is superior to other methods of control of computing functions and robotic vehicles. Promising areas for continued BMI research include the control of robotic orthotics and the management of information flow to an individual based on changes in the user's cognitive state.

Robotic Prostheses and Orthotics

Robotic prosthetics and orthotics are mechatronic systems that can be considered a form of assistive robotics. Prostheses replace a body part, and orthotic devices work in cooperation with the body, which helps to control them and/or assist in movement. While there are many applications for orthotic devices made for rehabilitative purposes (Krebs et al., 2004), focus is on devices that have been designed to improve or extend human performance in the physical domain.

Krebs et al. (2004, p. 353) observed that progress in the development of limb prostheses "has been modest. This may be partly due to irregular interest in their development, which tends to correlate with major wars." As a result, a 1991 survey estimated that "only 10% of prosthesis users in the U.S. (5% of the upper-limb amputee population) operate externally powered devices" (Krebs et al., 2004, p. 354). Until effective methods for EMG control, direct and natural feedback, and impedance control (e.g., for contact tasks) are developed, the adoption of externally powered artificial limbs will continue to be slow, although research continues on anatomically analogous model limbs with some success (Herr et al., 2003; Schwartz, 2004).

The problem of impedance control warrants further explanation. When a powered prosthesis under human control is designed to grasp an object, there must be feedback to the human for the amount of force that is being applied. The fact that some objects are soft and others hard means that it is not just information on the amount of force that must be fed back, but the force-compliance relationship as well—that is, how much the object is being squeezed to achieve a given amount of force. The human motor system normally manages this relationship unconsciously.

With respect to robotic orthotics, a variety of exoskeletons have been developed to increase human strength, endurance, and speed. It is difficult to say exactly what an exoskeleton is. To some extent, an automobile might be considered a kind of exoskeleton because it allows humans to move farther and faster and because the experience of driving can give the driver the feeling that the car is an extension of him or her self. The goal of research on orthotic exoskeletons is for the interface to be so transparent that there is no learning involved—the user simply performs the task in the usual way, and the system responds as if the wearer simply had stronger, faster, or more accurate limbs. This requires that the device do three things: (1) determine the user's intent, (2) apply forces when and where appropriate, and (3) get out of the way of the user's natural movement (Pratt et al., 2004). Examples of types of orthotic exoskeletons include mechanical interfaces to the upper body allowing a person to lift and move extremely heavy loads (Kazerooni, 1996) and devices interfacing with the lower extremities, allowing people to carry heavy loads for long periods of time or to cover long distances with minimal fatigue (Weiss, 2001; Kawamoto and Sonkai, 2002; Walsh et al., 2007). One such device, the RoboKnee, is an endurance multiplier. A user wearing a 60 kg backpack can do one-legged deep knee bends for an unlimited period of time, while without the device the user is limited to two or three such bends (Pratt et al., 2004). Concept designs have been advanced for biologically inspired exoskeletons that would significantly increase the speed and endurance of human divers (Neuhaus, 2004). While such designs are in their early stages of development, the potential advantages of biologically inspired approaches are considerable, including increased stealth (unlike propeller-driven devices, which produce a distinct signature, they are indistinguishable from background noise), natural interface (they form a transparent extension of the wearer's body), and hands-free operation (they can be operated using only the lower body). With today's components, a cruising speed of 1 m/sec is feasible with approximately 2.4 kg off-the-shelf silver-zinc batteries.

Some of the short-term technological challenges include reducing the various forms of impedance to the user's natural motion, increasing the comfort and naturalness of the interface so that users feel the exoskeleton is an extension of their body, making it easier to put on and take off the device, and increasing the length of time between recharges while making the batteries less bulky (Pratt et al., 2004). For swimming aids, challenges include the fabrication of materials that resist corrosion, are flexible and strong, and can be made reliably waterproof to protect electronic and mechanical components. See Figure 3-1 for an example of an exoskeleton.

Over the long term, there are hopes that advances in two key areas will make such devices more comfortable and practical: (1) replacing today's bulky actuators with artificial muscle (see, for example, Herr et al., 2003; Gordon and Ferris, 2007; Walsh et al., 2007) and (2) replacing current methods for determining user intent with direct BMIs. With respect to the first area, the important issues are not only power and force density but also low inherent impedance. Pratt et al. (2004) summarizes this very challenging problem and a possible approach as follows:

> Real muscle gets its low impedance since each actin-myosin pair is either engaged and force-producing or *completely disengaged*. Perhaps artificial muscle technology will need to operate on this physical principle of muscle in order to be useful for exoskeletons. . . . One can envision an artificial muscle on the micro or nano scale consisting of millions to billions of tiny latching devices, each with low impedance when producing force, and zero impedance when detached. Such actuators would also greatly reduce energy requirements for low-impedance motions.

Dennis and Herr (2005) document significant progress in materials for artificial muscles, with "electroactive polymers. . . rapidly emerging as quantitatively functional equivalents to muscle tissue, and it is likely that the technological evolution of EAP muscles will soon outpace the natural functional evolution of living muscle tissue." That having been said, they note significant advantages to natural muscle tissue in hybrid biomechatronic prosthetic systems and implants. With respect to user intent, Kawamoto and Sankai (2002) have investigated EMG-based

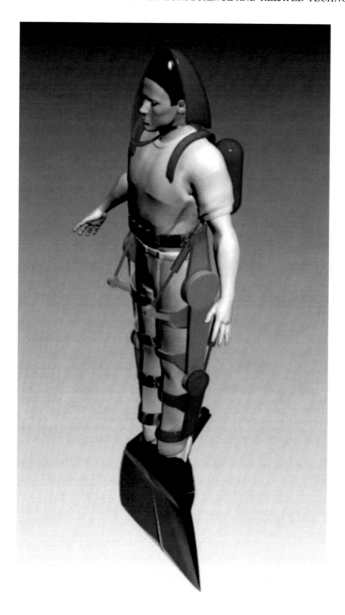

FIGURE 3-1 Example of a swimming exoskeleton. Such an exoskeleton not only has the potential of increasing the speed and range of a swimmer but can also increase stealth by mimicking fishlike rather than machinelike movement. SOURCE: Reprinted with permission from Peter Neuhaus and the Institute for Human and Machine Cognition at the University of West Florida.

commands with some success, building on the long interest in EMG control for upper-extremity motions (e.g., wrist rotations, grasping) (Krebs et al., 2004).

Finding 3-3. Research in robotic orthotics has produced a variety of exoskeletons to increase human strength, endurance, and speed. Challenges include the development of alternatives to today's bulky actuators (i.e., artificial muscle) and of appropriate BMIs for control and feedback.

Cognitive and Sensory Prostheses

These technologies aim to improve or extend human performance in the cognitive or sensory domain. Research in augmented cognition aims for closed-loop operation by continually sensing operator state and providing transparent augmentation of operator capabilities.

Boff (2006, p. 391) terms these developments Generation 3 of human factors and ergonomics (HFE):

> Generation 1 HFE evolved with a focus on *adapting* equipment, workplace, and tasks to human capabilities and limitations. Generation 2, focused on cognitive systems integration, arose in response to the need to manage automation and dynamic function allocation. Generation 3 is focused on the symbiotic technologies that can amplify human physical and cognitive capabilities. Generation 4 is emergent and is focused on biological enhancement of physical or cognitive capabilities.

Almost 50 years ago, the concept of "man–computer symbiosis" was introduced: "The hope is that, in not too many years, human brains and computing machines will be coupled together very tightly and that the resulting partnership will think as no human brain has ever thought and process data in a way not approached by the information-handling machines we know today" (Licklider, 1960, p. 4). The idea was something significantly more than a brain-machine interface—the goal was not merely to control external devices by interfacing them with the brain but to augment human cognitive and sensory abilities, directly improving human performance (Engelbart, 1962).

Eyeglasses, a well-known example of an ocular prosthesis, exemplify particularly well the three concepts that underlie cognitive and sensory prostheses (Ford et al., 1997):

• *Transparency.* "Eyeglasses leverage and extend our ability to see, but in no way model our eyes: They don't look or act like them and wouldn't pass a Turing test for being an eye" (Ford et al., 1997, p. 104). A key feature of eyeglasses is that they can be used more or less transparently—or, by forgetting they are present—just as humans with myopia don't think constantly about the wearing of the contact lenses but do know they are seeing more effectively *through* them.

• *Unity.* Since the goal is not to make smart eyeglasses but to improve an individual's ability to see, the design of the prosthesis must consider the device, the individual, and the environment in which the individual will use the device. This mode of analysis necessarily blurs the line between humans and technology.

• *Fit.* Your eyeglasses won't fit me; neither will mine do you any good. Prostheses must fit the human and technological components together in ways that synergistically exploit their mutual strengths and mitigate their respective limitations. This requires a rich knowledge of human function—of humans in general and of the particular individual being supported. A good example of this is the OZ cockpit display (Still and Temme, 2001). Through a groundbreaking study on the limits of human central and peripheral vision, Still discovered that peripheral vision can pick up an order of magnitude more detail than previously thought. Using this finding, he tailored the design of stimuli in a cockpit display to exploit the human sensory system's natural filtering and processing capabilities and to manipulate the data so they provide exactly what the pilot needs to know at any particular time. The result was a radically new approach where key data were represented in semantic primitives consistent across diverse types of aircraft. Stunningly, the OZ cockpit display (Figure 3-2) is devoid of the dials and gauges in ordinary cockpits yet easier to learn, more straightforward to control, and more robust to turbulent flight conditions and temporary visual system impairment.

The elaboration of foundational concepts for cognitive and robotic prostheses and the study of human functioning in particular environments happily dovetail with progress in the miniaturization of computing devices and the formulation of design principles for wearable computing. Mann was among the first to elucidate some of the criteria for devices to be successfully subsumed into the human being's eudemonistic space (the space where the device seems to be part of the person). He describes three required operational uses for wearable computing: constant readiness, augmentation of the intellect and/or senses, and mediation— meaning that the device can block out or alter reality (Mann, 1997). Figure 3-3 shows an example of visual prosthesis design for combat operations.

One domain where these concepts are being applied is "sensory substitution." Specific areas of the brain (e.g., the visual cortex) receive information from specific sensory organs (e.g., the eyes) in the form of pulses carried by afferent nerves. Sensory feedback from these organs associated with interaction with the environment guides and reinforces sensory perception. Sensory interfaces to an external system can consist of precisely positioned large magnetic fields (Kupers et al., 2006) or surgically implanted devices like cortical (Fernández et al., 2005) and end organ stimulators such as cochlear or retinal implants (Zhou and Greenberg, 2005), but this adds both surgical trauma and risk of infection (Reefhuis et al, 2003). Because perception takes place in the brain, not at the end organ (Bach-y-Rita, 1972; Bach-y-Rita et al., 2003), the brain can reinterpret sig-

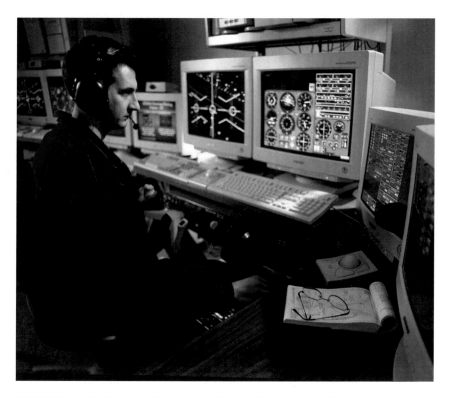

FIGURE 3-2 OZ display (left) versus traditional display (right). Due to the complexity of certification, such flight technologies will probably be applied first for the piloting of UAVs rather than manned aircraft. Intelligence analysts could use displays based on similar principles to allow them to process large amounts of information more reliably. SOURCE: Still and Temme (2001).

nals from specific nervous pathways (e.g., from tactile receptors) with appropriate sensory-motor feedback. This ability forms the basis for sensory substitution interfaces that use non-invasive and unobtrusive alternative sensory pathways to extend human sensory capabilities without interfering with existing sensory information processing (Bach-y-Rita and Kercel, 2003). Among the widely publicized examples of sensory substitution include projects designed to allow people to see with their ears (Motluk, 2005) and with their tongue (Bach-y-Rita et al., 1998; Nelson, 2006).

The characteristic of plasticity, inherent to the brain and the nervous system, supports both long-term and short-term anatomical and functional remapping of sensory data (Finkel, 1990; Walcott and Langdon, 2001), and researchers using sensory substitution interfaces for individuals with sensory loss due to

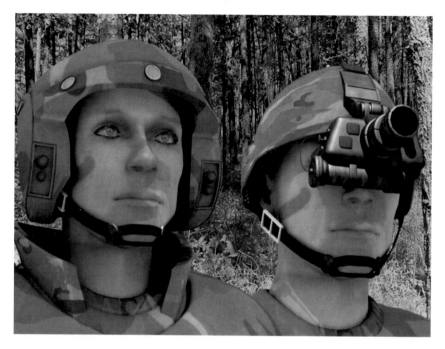

FIGURE 3-3 Visual prosthesis design for combat operations. Unlike current night vision systems (right), sensory substitution for night vision would not impede use of the eyes at night (left). SOURCE: Reprinted with permission from Anil Raj and the Institute for Human and Machine Cognition at the University of West Florida.

disease, congenital defect, or physical trauma have demonstrated enhancement of situation awareness (Ptito et al., 2005; Veraart et al., 2004; Kaczmarek et al., 1985; Saunders et al., 1981). Additionally, projections from visual, auditory, and proprioceptive sensory systems interact in the brain stem (Meredith and Stein, 1986a,b), indicating that the sensory channels operate cross-modally, possibly to reduce ambiguities in data sensed by single end-organ receptors. This provides a rationale for incorporating similar cross-modal techniques into multiple sensory channel substitution interfaces for the control of complex systems such as teleoperated robots, aircraft, and vehicles and is supported by adverse workload performance and situational awareness effects when veridical information is limited to a subset of normal sensory channels (Paivio, 1991; Wickens and Holland, 1999). Applications and approaches to sensory substitution through 2003 were cataloged by Lenay et al. (2003). Efforts to develop a comprehensive approach to the integration and dynamic adjustment of multi sensory input are described in Raj et al. (2000). Figure 3-4 illustrates a Vibrotactile displays for pilots.

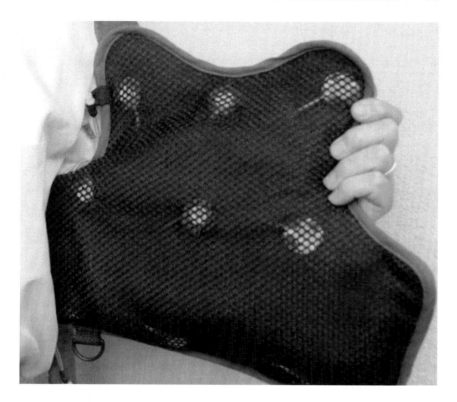

FIGURE 3-4 Vibrotactile displays for pilots experiencing sensory overload or cognitive illusions have been a successful application of sensory substitution technologies. Pilots, operators of complex equipment, and analysts monitoring large amounts of data can benefit as information is made available through underused sensory modalities that are more effective in some contexts than vision or hearing. SOURCE: Raj et al. (2005).

The Defense Advanced Research Projects Agency's (DARPA's) Augmented Cognition (AugCog) program was a research effort focused on appropriately exploiting and integrating all channels of communication from agents to humans (e.g., visual, auditory, tactile) and, conversely, sensing and interpreting a wide range of physiological measures of the human being in real time so they can be used to tune assistive behavior and thus enhance joint human-machine performance.[13] For example, sets of system sensor agents (say, a joystick), human sensor agents (EEG, pupil tracking, arousal meter), human display agents (visual, auditory, tactile), and adaptive automation agents (say, assisting in the perfor-

---

[13]For additional information, please see the Augmented Cognition International Society Web site at http://www.augmentedcognition.org. Last accessed on January 9, 2008.

mance of specific flight tasks) could work together with a pilot to promote stable and safe flight, sharing and adjusting aspects of control among the human and virtual crew member agents while taking system failures and human attention and stress loads into account.

Technologies developed for recent AugCog applications detect and classify human cognitive states such as fatigue, alertness decrement, inattention, or mental and sensory overload in real time by tracking changes in human behavioral and physiological patterns (Schmorrow and Kruse, 2004; Reeves et al., 2007). Using advanced machine learning algorithms, automated biosignal analyses have been developed (Trejo et al., 2003) that require as little as 3.5 sec of EEG data for a robust multivariate support vector classifier to correctly identify cognitive fatigue in 90 percent of individuals performing a demanding 3-hour task (Trejo et al., 2003, 2004).

To date most of the effort has gone into measuring "cognitive state," where gains have been made in the measurement of relatively simple constructs, but serious challenges have arisen in the measurement of complex cognitive constructs in real-world settings and in calibrating them to individual differences. While it is still too early to gauge the success of efforts such as AugCog, let alone to establish principles for making cognitive prostheses acceptable, it is clear that such advances will require new ways of thinking about human-machine interaction. A final note should be made about other forms of machine monitoring. These forms include real-time computer "reading" of human emotions (for example, optical recognition of facial expressions), of cognitive status (with, say, acoustic analyses of the voice), and of alertness/arousal (perhaps by optical tracking of slow eyelid closures [PERCLOS]). These capitalize on newer mathematical techniques such as active shape modeling, which has some potential. Figure 3-5 depicts a closed-loop augmented cognition concept of operation.

Finding 3-4. Researchers using sensory substitution interfaces in individuals with sensory loss have demonstrated enhanced situational awareness in their subjects. Thus use of similar cross-modal techniques with multiple sensory channel substitution interfaces shows promise for control of complex systems. Consistent with Finding 2-1, efforts in augmented cognition, which is sometimes oversold, have had some success in sensing and interpreting physiological measures of superordinate psychological states. These measures were calibrated to individuals in real time to tailor the assistive behavior and to manage information flow.

Software and Robotic Assistants

Many kinds of software and hardware (in the form of robotic assistants) are being designed in hope of improving or extending human performance in the physical and/or cognitive domains (Bradshaw, 1997; Lieberman, 2001; Murphy, 2000). However, they achieve their effect by interacting with the operator as

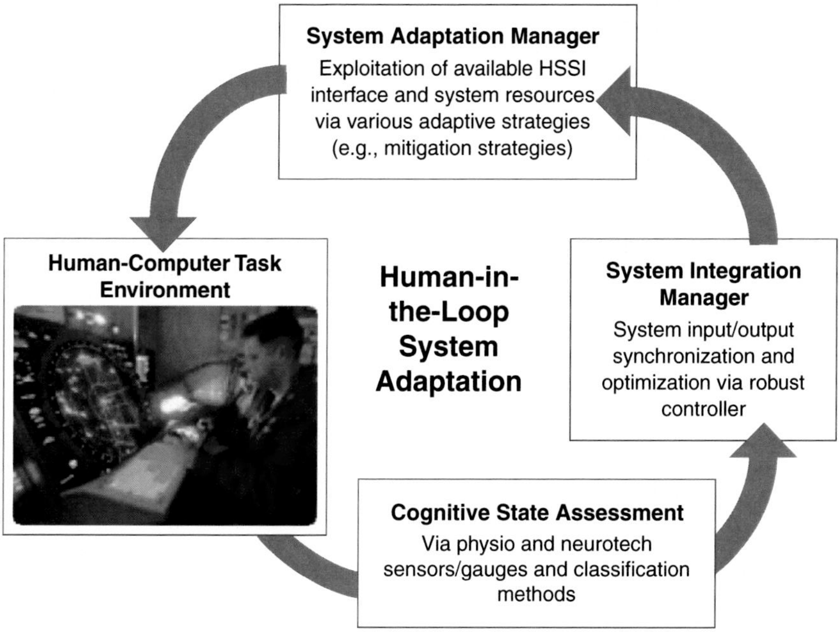

FIGURE 3-5 Closed-loop augmented cognition concept of operation. SOURCE: Schmorrow and Kruse (2004).

assistants or team members rather than to the body, brain, or senses to extend them. Software assistants can enable sophisticated forms of remote sensing, deliberation, and action in concert with humans and other assistants. Embedding a software assistant in a robot or unmanned vehicle provides the additional benefit of physical mobility.

Building an assistant might entail modeling the human brain. While modeling the whole brain is highly unlikely in the next two decades, it is not unreasonable to imagine that significant subsystems could be modeled. Moreover, it seems likely that increasingly sophisticated cognitive systems will be constructed in those two decades that, while not aiming to mimic processes in the brain, could nonetheless perform similar tasks well enough to be useful, especially in constrained situations. In this case, success would not be determined by how closely the system resembled the brain's mechanisms for action, but by how similar the performance of specific cognitive tasks was to a typical human user.

While a machine that simulates a complete human brain would be useful, it would be almost as useful to have high-performing machines simulating replicas of different cognitive capabilities. For example, a machine-enabled visual cortex could save untold hours of manual labor spent studying images from satellites or other sorts of reconnaissance photographs, in effect augmenting human performance. Although there are rudimentary systems for image detection through pattern recognition, scientists are still far from replacing live subject matter experts in this area. However, one can imagine an intelligent machine that not only recognizes patterns as well as an expert but also could do this over an entire spectrum of wavelengths that are inaccessible to the human eye. Similarly, one can also imagine a machine-based "ear" listening to radio communications and identifying crucial conversations. Research suggests that the combination of a robotic assistant and a human expert in pattern recognition, in which the robotic assistant automatically scans a photograph for areas that are likely to hold targets and directs the human to search again in those more likely areas, can improve detection probability and the efficiency of the search (see, for example, Oren et al., 2008; Mařík et al., 2008).

Research in artificial intelligence (AI) and cognitive science has pursued such objectives for many years, with reasonable success in many domains of understanding and application. Some AI researchers are focused on maximizing fidelity to cognitive neurophysiology, with the aim of increasing the scientific understanding of human functioning. Others are more concerned with the practical engineering of useful intelligent systems through an eclectic mix of engineering know-how and an understanding of human intelligence. Yet others wish to enhance human performance by combining the strengths of humans and automation. Success over the next two decades will require an appreciation of all perspectives, neither undervaluing the independent study of human functioning nor slavishly imitating superfluous aspects of natural systems in the development of artificial ones, like the engineer who insists that airplanes must have flapping wings because birds have them (Ford and Hayes, 1998).

Making up in part for a lack of "experience" on which much of human expertise is based, intelligent systems are increasingly using the Internet, now the largest repository of knowledge on the planet, to learn. By way of contrast, early intelligent systems were like the disembodied brains shown in low-budget science fiction movies: entities that ruled the world while floating in a glass jar tethered by wires. While potentially rich in internal knowledge and inferential power, their only direct experience of the world arrived through the impoverished modes of keyboard input and video display output. The Internet's rise and the multitude of specialized interactive devices it has spawned give intelligent systems rich means to sense, learn, and interact with humans and within cyberspace. Because this sort of intelligence is distributed, coordination becomes as important as cognition. Thus many researchers have increasingly abandoned the metaphor of the intelligent system as disembodied brain in favor of that of the agent as software robot. This research emphasis has subtly shifted much of the newer research from deliberation to doing, from reasoning to remote action.

There are no fundamental reasons why artificial cognitive systems designed for specific functions could not be constructed. Such systems could employ reusable software components to embody the "intelligence" needed for specific human tasks. The main practical limitation, other than memory and processing power, is coming up with more powerful and efficient means of drawing conclusions from these data. There is reason to believe that if science has not yet met the technical specifications for an artificial cognitive system, it will certainly do so in the near future. With only modest research funding, surprise breakthroughs in this area could come not only from the United States but also from any one of a number of countries in Europe or Asia in the coming 10 years.

In contrast to research that has focused on how to increase the autonomy of intelligent systems, efforts are under way to better understand and satisfy requirements for software and robotic assistants that can work in close and continuous collaboration with people. The considerable interdependence of humans and machines in such applications requires that, in addition to what people and assistants do to accomplish the work itself, they must also invest time and attention to making sure that their tasks are appropriately coordinated. Through the effective handling of these concerns, human attention can remain focused on critical tasks, costly errors can be avoided, and individual and group performance can be significantly enhanced.

There are many potential military and intelligence applications of software assistants in the form of software and robots. Promising areas include the following (Bradshaw et al., 2003):

• PLOW is a good example of a state-of-the-art software assistant that helps people manage their everyday tasks (Allen et al., 2007). It uses the same collaborative architecture to learn tasks as it does to perform tasks. PLOW displays an intelligence that springs from sophisticated natural language understanding, reasoning, learning, and acting capabilities unified within a collaborative agent architecture.

• Robotic assistants respond to the growing use of unmanned systems in the military, whereby large numbers of heterogeneous unmanned ground, air, underwater, and surface vehicles work together, coordinated by a smaller number of human operators (Summey et al., 2001). A key requirement for such systems is real-time cooperation with people and with other autonomous systems (Goodrich and Schultz, 2007). While these heterogeneous cooperating platforms may operate at different levels of sophistication and with dynamically varying degrees of autonomy, they will require some common means of representing and appropriately participating in joint tasks. Just as important, developers of such systems will need tools and methodologies to assure that the systems work together reliably and safely even when they are designed independently.

"Teamwork" is a widely accepted term for describing the cooperation among people and intelligent systems (Tambe et al., 1999; Klein et al., 2004). The idea is that shared knowledge, goals, and intentions are a glue that binds team members together. By having a largely reusable explicit formal model of shared intentions, team members attempt to manage general responsibilities and commitments to each other in a coherent fashion that facilitates recovery when unanticipated problems arise. For example, it often happens in joint action that one team member fails and can no longer perform. A teamwork model might stipulate that each team member be notified, under appropriate conditions, of the failure, thus reducing the requirement for special-purpose, exception-handling mechanisms for each possible failure mode (Cohen and Levesque, 1991).

Finding 3-5. Software and robotic assistants are designed to improve or extend human performance in the physical and cognitive domains. Much of the newer research has shifted from deliberation to doing, from reasoning to acting remotely. This suggests a blurring of discipline boundaries such that new indicators and observables are needed. Progress will require investments in the development of (1) reusable software components that embody the intelligence needed to support specific human tasks and (2) assistants that can coordinate their interaction with humans and artificial assistants in ways that emulate natural and effective teamwork within groups of people.

Finding 3-6. As high-performance computing becomes less expensive and more available, a country could become a world leader in cognitive neuroscience through sustained investment in the nurture of local talent and the construction of required infrastructure. Key to allowing breakthroughs will be the development of software-based models and algorithms, areas in which much of the world is now on par with or ahead of the United States. Given the proliferation of highly skilled software researchers around the world and the relatively low cost of establishing and sustaining the necessary organizational infrastructure in many other countries, the United States cannot expect to easily maintain its technical superiority.

Recommendation 3-1. The intelligence community, in collaboration with outside experts, should develop the capability to monitor international progress and investments in computational neuroscience. Particular attention should be given to countries where software research and development are relatively inexpensive and where there exists a sizeable workforce with the appropriate education and skills.

Finding 3-7. Unlike in the domain of cognitive neurophysiological research, where the topics are constrained by certain aspects of human physiology and brain functioning, progress in the domain of artificial cognitive systems and distributed human-machine systems (DHMS) is limited only by the creative imagination. Accordingly, with sustained scientific leadership there is reason for optimism about the continued development of (1) specialized artificial cognitive systems that emulate specific aspects of human performance and (2) DHMS, whether through approaches that are faithful to cognitive neurophysiology, or through some mix of engineering and studies of human intelligence, or by combining the respective strengths of humans and automation working in concert. Researchers are addressing the limitations that made earlier systems brittle by exploring ways to combine human and machine capabilities to solve problems and by modeling coordination and teamwork as an essential aspect of system design.

Research in artificial cognitive systems and DHMS faces two problems. One is the unrealistic programs driven by the specific, short-term needs of DoD and the intelligence community. The second problem is the inadequacy of the current approach to metric measurement systems, which makes it next to impossible to achieve meaningful progress because it deals chiefly with epiphenomena of limited value.

REFERENCES

Allen, J., N. Chambers, G. Ferguson, L. Galescu, H. Jung, M. Swift, and W. Taysom. 2007. PLOW: A collaborative task learning agent. In *Proceedings of Association for the Advancement of Artificial Intelligence (AAAI) 2007*. Vancouver, British Columbia: AAAI.

Bach-y-Rita, Paul. 1972. *Brain Mechanisms in Sensory Substitution*. New York: Academic Press.

Bach-y-Rita, Paul. 1996. Nonsynaptic diffusion neurotransmission and brain plasticity. *The Neuroscientist* 2(5):260-261.

Bach-y-Rita, P., and S.W. Kercel. 2003. Sensory substitution and the human-machine interface. *Trends in Cognitive Sciences* 7(12):541-546.

Bach-y-Rita, P., K. Kaczmarek, M. Tyler, and J. Garcia-Lara. 1998. Form perception with a 49-point electrotactile stimulus array on the tongue. *Journal of Rehabilitation Research Development* 35(4):427-430.

Bach-y-Rita, P., M.E. Tyler, and K.A. Kaczmarek. 2003. Seeing with the brain. *International Journal of Human-Computer Interaction* 15(2):287-297.

Birbaumer, Niels. 2006. Breaking the silence: Brain-computer interfaces (BCI) for communication and motor control. *Psychophysiology* 43(6):517-532.

Birbaumer, Niels. 2007. Brain-computer interfaces: Communication and restoration of movement in paralysis. *Journal of Physiology* 579(3):621-636.

Boff, Kenneth R. 2006. Revolutions and shifting paradigms in human factors and ergonomics. *Applied Ergonomics* 37(4; July):391-399. Special Issue: Meeting Diversity in Ergonomics.

Bradshaw, Jeffery M., ed. 1997. *Software Agents*. Cambridge, MA: AAAI Press/MIT Press.

Bradshaw, J.M., G. Boy, E. Durfee, M. Gruninger, H. Hexmoor, N. Suri, M. Tambe, M. Uschold, and J. Vitek, eds. 2003. Software agents for the warfighter. *ITAC Consortium Report*. Cambridge, MA: AAAI Press/The MIT Press.

Cohen, P.R., and H.J. Levesque. 1991. *Teamwork*. Menlo Park, CA: SRI International.

Dennis, R.G., and H. Herr. 2005. Engineered muscle actuators: Cells and tissues. Pp. 243-266 in *Biomimetics: Biologically Inspired Technologies*, Y. Bar-Cohen, ed. Boca Raton, FL: CRC Press.

DiGiovanna, J., B. Mahmoudi, J. Mitzelfelt, J.C. Sanchez, and J.C. Principe. 2007. Brain-machine interface control via reinforcement learning. Pp. 530-533 in *3rd International IEEE/EMBS Conference on Neural Engineering, CNE '07*, May 2-5, Kohala Coast, HI.

Drabløs, Finn, Mikael Hammer, Astrid Lægreid, Jon Olav Hauglid, and Bjørn K. Alsberg. 2004. Bio-informatics towards 2020. Paper read at the Information Society of 2020 (InfoSam2020) conference, April 19-20, Trondheim, Norway. Available from https://www.ime.ntnu.no/infosam2020/oldpage/Conference/Conference_Papers_2ndEdition_2.pdf. Last accessed June 18, 2008.

Engelbart, D.C. 1962. *Augmenting Human Intellect: A Conceptual Framework.* Menlo Park, CA: Stanford Research Institute.

Fernández, E., F. Pelayo, S. Romero, M. Bongard, C. Marin, A. Alfaro, and L. Merabet. 2005. Development of a cortical visual neuroprosthesis for the blind: The relevance of neuroplasticity. *Journal of Neural Engineering* 2(4):R1-12.

Finkel, L.H. 1990. A model of receptive field plasticity and topographic map reorganization in the somatosensory cortex. Pp. 164-192 in *Connectionist Modeling and Brain Function: The Developing Interface*, S.J. Hanson and C.R. Olsen, eds. Cambridge, MA: MIT Press.

Ford, K.M., C. Glymour, and P. Hayes. 1997. Cognitive prostheses. *AI Magazine* 18(3):104.

Ford, K.M., and P. Hayes. 1998. On computational wings: Rethinking the goals of artificial intelligence. *Scientific American. Special Issue, "Exploring Intelligence,"* 9(4):78-83.

Goldstein, Jeffrey. 1999. Emergence as a construct: History and issues. *Emergence: Complexity and Organization* 1:49-72.

Goodrich, M.A., and A.C. Schultz. 2007. Human-robot interaction: A survey. *Foundations and Trends in Human-Computer Interaction* 1(3):203-275.

Gordon, K.E., and D.P. Ferris. 2007. Learning to walk with a robotic ankle exoskeleton. *Journal of Biomechanics* 40(12):2636-2644.

Herr, H., G. Whiteley, and D. Childress. 2003. Cyborg technology—biomimetic orthotic and prosthetic technology. Pp. 103-144 in *Biologically Inspired Intelligent Robots*, Y. Bar-Cohen and C. Breazeal, eds. Bellingham, WA.: SPIE Press.

Kaczmarek, K., P. Bach-y-Rita, W.J. Tompkins, and J.G. Webster. 1985. A tactile vision-substitution system for the blind: Computer-controlled partial image sequencing. *IEEE Transactions on Biomedical Engineering* BME-32:602-608.

Kawamoto, H., and Y. Sankai. 2002. Comfortable power assist control method for walking aid by HAL-3. In *Proceedings of the IEEE International Conference on Systems, Man and Cybernetics*, Vol. 4. October 6-9, Yasmine Hammamet, Tunisia.

Kazerooni, H. 1996. The human power amplifier technology at the University of California, Berkeley. *Journal of Robotics and Autonomous Systems* 19:179-187.

Klein, G., P.J. Feltovich, J.M. Bradshaw, and D.D. Woods. 2004. Common ground and coordination in joint activity. Pp. 139-184 in *Organizational Simulation*, Vol. 1, W.B. Rouse and K.R. Boff, eds. New York, NY: John Wiley.

Krebs, H.I., N. Hogan, W. Durfee, and H. Herr. 2004. Rehabilitation robotics, orthotics, and prosthetics. Pp. 337-369 in *Textbook of Neural Repair and Rehabilitation*, Vol. 1, M.E. Selzer, S. Clarke, L.G. Cohen, P.W. Duncan, and F.H. Gage, eds. Cambridge, England: Cambridge University Press.

Kupers R., A. Fumal, A.M. de Noordhout, A. Gjedde, J. Schoenen, and M. Ptito. 2006. Transcranial magnetic stimulation of the visual cortex induces somatotopically organized qualia in blind subjects. *Proceedings of the National Academy of Sciences U.S.A.* 103(35):13256-13260.

Lenay, C., O. Gapenne, S. Hanneton, C. Genouëlle, and C. Marque. 2003. Sensory substitution, limits and perspectives. In *Touching for Knowing: Cognitive Psychology of Haptic Manual*, Y. Hatwell, A. Streri, and E. Gentaz, eds. Available from http://www.utc.fr/gsp/publi/Lenay03-SensorySubstitution.pdf. Last accessed on February 11, 2008.

Licklider, J.C.R. 1960. Man-computer symbiosis. *IRE Transactions on Human Factors in Electronics* HFE-1(2):4-11.

Lieberman, H., ed. 2001. *Your Wish Is My Command: Programming by Example.* San Francisco: Morgan Kaufmann Publishers.

Mann, S. 1997. Wearable computing: A first step toward personal imaging. *IEEE Computer* 30(2):25-32.

Mařík, V., J.M. Bradshaw, J. Meyer, W.A. Gruver, and Petr Benda. 2008. Pp. 63-68 in *Proceedings of the 2008 IEEE International Conference on Distributed Human-Machine Systems (DHMS 2008)*. March 9-12, Athens, Greece.

Meredith, M.A., and B.E. Stein. 1986a. Spatial factors determine the activity of multisensory neurons in cat superior colliculus. *Brain Research* 365(2):350-354.

Meredith, M.A. and B.E. Stein. 1986b. Visual, auditory, and somatosensory convergence on cells in superior colliculus results in multisensory integration. *Journal of Neurophysiology* 56(3):640-662.

Motluk, A. Seeing with your ears. *The New York Times* Online Edition, December 11, 2005. Available from http://www.nytimes.com/2005/12/11/magazine/11ideas_section3-14.html?ex=1291957200&en=3c72cf9fa46bbb06&ei=5090&partner=rssuserland&emc=rss. Last accessed June 18, 2008.

Murphy, R.R. 2000. *Introduction to AI Robotics*. Cambridge, MA: The MIT Press.

Nelson, M. 2006. Scientists probe use of the tongue. *USA Today* Online, April 24, 2006. Available from http://www.usatoday.com/tech/science/discoveries/2006-04-24-tongue-research_x.htm. Last accessed June 18, 2008.

Ng, Lydia, Sayan Pathak, Chihchau Kuan, Chris Lau, Hong-wei Dong, Andrew Sodt, Chinh Dang, Brian Avants, Paul Yushkevich, James Gee, David Haynor, Ed Lein, Allan Jones, and Mike Hawrylycz. 2007. Neuroinformatics for genome-wide 3-D gene expression mapping in the mouse brain. *IEEE/ACM Transactions on Computational Biology and Bioinformatics* 4(3):382-393.

Oren, Y, A. Bechar, J. Meyer, and Y. Edan. 2008. Performance analysis of human-robot collaboration in target recognition tasks. Paper read at IEEE International Conference on Distributed Human-Machine Systems (DHMS 2008), Athens, Greece, March 9-12, 2008.

Paivio, A. 1991. Dual coding theory: Retrospect and current status. *Canadian Journal of Psychology* 45(3):255-287.

Pratt, J.E., B.T. Krupp, C.J. Morse, and S.H. Collins. 2004. The RoboKnee: An exoskeleton for enhancing strength and endurance during walking. Pp. 2430-2435 in *Proceedings of the 2004 IEEE International Conference on Robotics and Automation,* Vol. 3. New Orleans, LA. April 26-May 1.

Ptito, M., S.M. Moesgaard, A. Gjedde, and R. Kupers. 2005. Cross-modal plasticity revealed by electrotactile stimulation of the tongue in the congenitally blind. *Brain* 128(3):606-614.

Raj, A.K., S.J. Kass, and J.F. Perry. 2000. Vibrotactile displays for improving spatial awareness. In *Proceedings of the Human Factors and Ergonomics Society Annual Meeting* 1(4):181-184.

Raj, A.K., R.W. Carff, M.J. Johnson, S.P. Kulkarni, J.H. Higgins; and J.M. Bradshaw. 2005. A multi-sensory integrated representation architecture for notional display applications (MIRANDA). *Proceedings of the 1st International Conference on Virtual Reality*, Paper #86 on CD of Vol. 9, Advances in Virtual Environments Technology: Musings on Design, Evaluation, and Application. Mahwah, NJ: Lawrence Erlbaum Associates.

Reefhuis, Jennita, Margaret A. Honein, Cynthia G. Whitney, Shadi Chamany, Eric A. Mann, Krista R. Biernath, Karen Broder, Susan Manning, Swati Avashia, Marcia Victor, Pamela Costa, Owen Devine, Ann Graham, and Coleen Boyle. 2003. Risk of bacterial meningitis in children with cochlear implants. *New England Journal of Medicine* 349(5):435-445.

Reeves, L.M., D.D. Schmorrow, and K.M. Stanney. 2007. Augmented cognition and cognitive state assessment technology: Near-term, mid-term, and long-term research objectives. In LNAI 4565, *Foundations of Augmented Cognition,* D.D. Schmorrow and L.M. Reeves, eds. Berlin: Springer.

Saunders, F.A.,W.A. Hill, and B. Franklin. 1981. A wearable tactile sensory aid for profoundly deaf children. *Journal of Medical Systems* 5(4):265-270.

Schmorrow, D.D., and A.A. Kruse. 2004. Augmented cognition. Pp. 54-59 in *Berkshire Encyclopedia of Human-Computer Interaction*, W.S. Bainbridge, ed. Great Barrington, MA: Berkshire Publishing Group.

Schwartz, A.B. 2004. Cortical neural prosthetics. *Annual Review of Neurosciences* 27: 487-507.

Silver, Rae, Kwabena Boahen, Sten Grillner, Nancy Kopell, and Kathie L. Olsen. 2007. Neurotech for neuroscience: Unifying concepts, organizing principles, and emerging tools. *Journal of Neuroscience* 27(44):11807-11819.

Still, D.L., and L.A. Temme. 2001. OZ: A human-centered cockpit display. Paper read at the Interservice/Industry Training, Simulation, and Education Conference, Orlando, FL, November 26-29, 2001.

Summey, D.C., R.R. Rodrigues, D.P. DeMartino, H.H. Portmann Jr., and E. Moritz. 2001. *Shaping the Future of Naval Warfare with Unmanned Systems*. Panama City, FL: Dahlgren Division, Naval Surface Warfare Center.

Tambe, M., W. Shen, M. Mataric, D.V. Pynadath, D. Goldberg, P.J. Modi, Z. Qiu, and B. Salemi. 1999. Teamwork in cyberspace: Using TEAMCORE to make agents team-ready. Presented at AAAI Spring Symposium on Agents in Cyberspace, Menlo Park, CA. Available from http://www.isi.edu/~modi/papers/aaai-spring99.ps. Last accessed June 18, 2008.

Thomas, J.J., and K.A. Cook. 2005. Illuminating the path: The research and development agenda for visual analytics. Richland, WA: National Visualization and Analytics Center. Available from http://nvac.pnl.gov/agenda.stm#book. Last accessed January 10, 2008.

Trejo, L.J., K.R. Wheeler, C.C. Jorgensen, R. Rosipal, S. Clanton, B. Matthews, A.D. Hibbs, R. Matthews, and M. Krupka. 2003. Multimodal neuroelectric interface development. *IEEE Transactions on Neural Systems and Rehabilitation Engineering* 11(2):199-204.

Trejo, L.J., R. Kochavi, K. Kubitz, L.D. Montgomery, R. Rosipal, and B. Matthews. 2004. Measures and models for estimating and predicting cognitive fatigue. *Psychophysiology* 41:S86.

Veraart, C., F. Duret, M. Brelén, M. Oozeer, and J. Delbeke. 2004. Vision rehabilitation in the case of blindness. *Expert Review of Medical Devices* 1(1):139-153.

Walcott, E.C., and R.B. Langdon. 2001. Short-term plasticity of extrinsic excitatory inputs to neocortical layer 1. *Experimental Brain Research* 136(2):143-151.

Walsh, C.J., K. Endo, and H. Herr. 2007. A quasi-passive leg exoskeleton for load-carrying augmentation. *International Journal of Humanoid Robotics* 4(3):487-506.

Weiss, P. 2001. Dances with robots. *Science News* 159(26):407.

Wickens, C.D., and J. Holland. 1999. *Engineering Psychology and Human Performance,* 3rd Edition. Upper Saddle River, NJ: Prentice Hall, Inc.

Zhou, D., and R. Greenberg. 2005. Microsensors and microbiosensors for retinal implants. *Frontiers in Bioscience* 10(1):166-179.

4

Cultural and Ethical Underpinnings of Social Neuroscience

INTRODUCTION

In this chapter, the committee places the evolution of emerging cognitive neuroscience and related technologies in context by discussing the cultural and ethical issues associated with the science and technology. This discussion shows that advances in science and technology are not isolated in a laboratory and that the ways in which different cultures view the issues surrounding cognitive neuroscience are meaningful.

CULTURAL UNDERPINNINGS OF SOCIAL NEUROSCIENCE

Introduction

This section identifies trends in basic and applied social-science research on culture that can improve the U.S. intelligence community's (IC's) understanding of the expected directions of this research in the next 20 years.[1] In the context of the present report, this chapter serves as a link between scientific findings in neuroscience in general and current social-science research on culture in particular. The chapter also builds on the recommendation of a recent National Research Council report, *Human Behavior in Military Contexts,* that the military and the IC support several fields of relevant social-science research (NRC, 2008):

---

[1] For purposes of this report, "culture" is defined as a collective identity whose shared membership has distinct values, attitudes, and beliefs. Behavioral norms, practices, and rituals distinguish one cultural group from another. Distinct cultural groups are defined around regional, political, economic, ethnic, social, generational, or religious values.

it addresses how research on culture can advance effective intercultural competence, nonverbal behavior and emotion detection, and human, social, cultural, and behavioral models in national-security and military settings.

The problems facing national-security analysts will be discussed first. By definition, *culture* applies not only to nation-states but to individuals, ethnic groups, and transnational affiliates. Globalization requires national-security analysis to account more than ever for the political, social, economic, and cultural interactions, interests, and identities among states and especially nonstate actors. Contemporary foreign and military policy and intelligence gathering and analysis require understanding of the efforts undertaken by states in their dealings not only with other states but with numerous other external actors. Political realists in international relations have traditionally considered the state to be the most important element of concern. However, this chapter will begin with a discussion that shows that the selection of the unit of cultural analysis for understanding must be based on plural and global paradigms, not on political theory alone.

The array of research in political science; cultural anthropology; social, political, and cognitive psychology; and social neuroscience that is exploring implications of culture for cognition, meaning, and behavior will then be discussed. There are valid frameworks for assessing the values, preferences, and norms of cultural groups. The second part will outline the basic research and applied frameworks used to understand the cultural perspectives and mindset of individuals and of particular national cultures.

The third area of discussion will address whether research has shown that people can read, influence, or control the minds of others in various cultural and national contexts. Is brain functioning or neural mapping biologically universal, or is it culturally determined? It may not yet be possible to read minds with neuroscientific diagnostics and devices, but have practices in trust-building and management of fear that have relevance for the IC been developed in intercultural communication and conflict resolution? Conclusions will be drawn on how cultural research and frameworks can increase the effectiveness of programs in human behavior and culture models—such as the Human Terrain Project, GlobeSmart Soldier, and CultureSpan—under development by the IC and the military and diplomatic communities.

Culture and the Unit of Analysis

The study of culture requires a definition of the boundaries such as norms and ethics that identify a particular group. Political realism asserts that geographic and legal definitions of the state have been the bases of political and cultural understanding and interaction. Political realism has traditionally assumed that the state is a unitary actor (sometimes referred to as a black box) that has one policy or perspective at any given time on any particular issue. The state is essentially a legal and rational actor, which pursues foreign-policy and military-policy decision-making processes through consideration of all feasible alternatives and objectives and ultimately selects one that maximizes the security of the state. Political realism also assumes that national security is at the top of the list of issues that dominate world politics. Conflicts between states are maintained and addressed by using force to resolve disputes and prevent territorial violations (Viotti and Kauppi, 1987).

Pluralism uses a different set of assumptions. Whereas a nation is strictly defined as a group of people who have a common identity, states are often comprised of more than one nationality. Nonstate actors are critically important in international relations. International organizations and transnational corporations and affiliations, with their own organizational and ethnic cultural perspectives, have increasing influence on foreign and military policy. That challenges the notion that the state is a unitary actor but that it is composed of interest groups, bureaucracies, and individuals that have their own cultural identities and influences on foreign and military policy. The pursuit of individual cultural-value–maximizing strategies at an organizational level can lead to disaster or bias for state military or foreign policy. The pluralist paradigm rejects the notion that primarily military-security issues dominate the agenda of world politics. Economic, social, and cultural issues—not military ones—are often at the forefront of international affairs (Viotti and Kauppi, 1987).

The globalist view, which is fundamentally different from the realist and pluralist views, is that the global context within which states and other actors interact is important. Globalists emphasize the overall interdependent structure of international conditions and believe that actors are predisposed to behave in particular ways. States, societies, ethnic groups, and other nonstate actors operate as part of the entire world system. The globalist focus is on patterns of dominance within and among societies with respect to complex, and often conflicting, perspectives on economic, social, cultural, and political factors. In this view, national-security issues are dominated by groups that share transnational identities and interests but are often not bounded by a legal, sovereign-state, or by sanctioned foreign policy (Viotti and Kauppi, 1987).

Increasing global interdependence implies that societies and cultures will be brought into greater contact with one another (Friedman, 2005). Efforts to use social and cultural modeling and frameworks to predict behavior and intentions in an intelligence and military context will require a focus on the various patterns of organization of cultural groups. The IC's understanding of culture will be enhanced by a pluralist and globalist view of how culture groups are organized and how research is conducted and applied in the field of culture studies.

Need for Cultural Due Diligence

Cultural due diligence has traditionally included attention to communication and language systems, jargon, gestures, and dialects used to distinguish national cultural groups. Understanding of dress and appearance, food and dining habits, attitudes toward time, relationships, protocol, traditions, rituals, and greeting issues has become central in the effectiveness of interactions with national groups other than one's own (Harris et al., 2004). Lack of cultural attention can lead to embarrassing or even dangerous situations. In Iraq, the United States military misunderstood the system of information transmission in Iraqi society and consequently lost opportunities to influence public opinion (McFate, 2005).

Much of intercultural training and profiling has been on the protocol, gestures, greetings, and other observable behaviors that may differ among cultures. However, there has recently been more research on what "lies beneath the surface" of awareness and the internal world at the cognitive and emotional levels. Efforts are being made to understand better how behavior is linked to ideas and emotional values in the subconscious mind (the "bottom of the iceberg"). That is the new frontier of social neuroscience, and it links behavior with brain functioning, cognition, and emotions. Many contributors to the field of intercultural studies have analyzed cultural differences by state, but an increasingly pluralist and globalist view is being taken in the study of culture. National profiling is the easiest and most pragmatic way to differentiate distinct cultures (Dahl, 2000).

Within national groups there are often subgroups that have characteristics that distinguish them from others. Age, sex, social class, race, and sects can define the subgroups. The Arab-Muslim world, for example, is a vast, diverse civilization, "encompassing over one billion people and stretching from Morocco to Indonesia and from Nigeria to London. It is very dangerous to generalize about such a complex religious community, made of many different ethnicities and nationalities" (Friedman, 2005).

A pluralist view of culture would pay attention to the interrelated levels of culture, which are more practical for understanding human behavior. For the pluralist and globalist, the narrow focus on national culture is too simplistic for the social, political, and organizational complexity of the 21st century. Schmitz (2005), for example, asserts that it is possible to distinguish five interrelated levels of culture:

• *Interpersonal level*—the primary building block of culture. This is the level where culture is experienced and created through social interaction. Individuals are the reflections of a societal pattern of values and norms, and they cause cultural changes through active shifts and changes in these social patterns. An example is the interactions of the typical U.S. soldier stationed in Iraq or Afghanistan with Iraqis or Afghanis. Likewise, there are differences between one intelligence analyst who is schooled in the cultures of a foreign country and another who is a second-generation member of that very nationality or subnationality.
• *Group or team level*—refers to social, functional, or professional groups. Each group requires a set of values and norms if it is to be cohesive. As interactions shape the group dynamics, individuals directly affect the pattern of group values

and norms. Within the federal government, examples of these differences have long existed between the various uniformed services, as well as between the Central Intelligence Agency (CIA) and the Federal Bureau of Investigation (FBI).

• *Functional level*—describes the dominant values, norms, and practices that exist within a particular professional function. These are the patterns that characterize and distinguish, for example, human resources, marketing, operations, bureaucratic units, and legislative units. In the IC, examples of these include the differences in the CIA between Directorate of Intelligence analysts and their Directorate of Operations case-officer counterparts in the clandestine service.

• *Organizational level*—represents the deep patterns of values and norms that define societal institutions. Examples of these include the differences in the national-security realm between the uniformed services and the civilians, or between the Executive and the Legislative branches.

• *Societal or national level*—involves the distinctive set of values, norms, practices, and institutions that defines what it means to be a member of a society. The nation-state has been the most common form of this level of analysis that has primarily been addressed thus far in this chapter.

Each distinguishable cultural group is characterized by a distinct set of behavioral norms, practices, and institutions that define what it means to be a member of the group. Within each group, there will often be some variation around the dominant set of values, variation that is necessary if the group is to be able to adapt and change. These cultural groupings can identify the set of behavioral norms, practices, and institutions that guide particular cultures' members and overcomes the reductionist approach that compares cultures only in terms of their behavioral norms. The use of behavioral norms, practices, and institutions and a comparison model of cultural preferences can lend practical guidance in self-awareness and awareness of others (Walker et al., 2003).

Culture is understood to exist at all those interrelated levels and can be defined as the pattern of ideas, emotions, and observable manifestations (including behaviors, practices, institutions, and artifacts) that tends to be expected, reinforced, and rewarded by, and within, a particular group (Walker et al., 2003). Cultural-orientation models (COMs) are now used not only at the national level but as tools to describe, analyze, and facilitate interactions in any interpersonal, social, organizational, economic, or political cultural group.

Intercultural competence includes analysis of one's own cultural preferences, values, attitudes, and beliefs and of how they are reflected in one's behavior. Much of intercultural development and training builds on awareness of one's own culture and how that culture can lead to misunderstandings and destructive interactions with those in other cultural groups. Cultural knowledge is understood to be about not only a general knowledge of a cultural group but how life and values have been shaped by history. For example, a cultural analysis involves a focus on how conflicts have been solved, how decisions are made, and how people have been motivated and rewarded.

Cultural due diligence also includes assessing and preparing for a multi-cultural setting. It involves investigating the cultural backgrounds and orientations of members of a group and evaluating the potential and actual cultural differences by using the COM-like frameworks. One example is the GlobeSmart Commander used for training North Atlantic Treaty Organization multinational peacekeeping forces, and another is the GlobeSmart Soldier used in Iraq programs. Those programs involve training and development for U.S. military personnel through self-assessment surveys, gap analysis, briefings on culture and history, and cultural scenario exercises (Aperian Global, 2007).

Strategies and skills for minimizing adverse social effects must be developed. The idea is to know how one's own experiences and those of other cultures affect the perspective, outlook, and outcome to be achieved. One key skill involves style-switching; that is, developing the ability to use a broad and flexible behavioral repertoire to accomplish one's goals. Another key skill is to develop cultural dialogue abilities to elicit cultural information, to build trust and rapport through conversation, to illuminate cultural underpinnings of behavior and performance, and to close cultural gaps and create cultural synergy (Schmitz, 2005). This synergy builds on similarities and fuses differences, and the results are more effective human activities and systems (Harris et al., 2004). More than observation, conversation is a powerful means to reach new understandings and a new basis on which to think and act. These processes not only can elicit information but can lead to solving problems. Cultural mentoring, or assistance in facilitating cultural understanding and integration into new and different cultural environments, has become a demanding practice (Schmitz, 2005).

Other intercultural competences are the ability to communicate with someone in a way that does not offend or break rules, effectiveness when there is high anxiety and uncertainty, adaptation and adjustment in unfamiliar or dangerous surroundings, understanding of nonverbal and other types of face-saving and face-threatening strategies, mindfulness or openness to new information, and awareness of others' emotional states (Rudd and Lawson, 2007). Culturally competent negotiators, for example, rarely use lie-detection tools, such as polygraphy or other technology, but they do rely on due diligence to achieve a high level of business intelligence, and they use emotional, cultural, and social profiling to verify "signals" in a multicultural negotiation.

Cultural intelligence means being skilled and flexible in understanding a culture and learning how to reshape one's own thinking about interactions with people of other cultures (Thomas and Inksen, 2004). Like other forms of intelligence—such as social intelligence (the capacity to interact with and influence others) and emotional intelligence (the ability to regulate and use one's emotions)—cultural intelligence has become a subject of social-science research. For example, psychometric tools have been designed to measure the components of a global mind-set, which affects performance, influence, and effective behaviors in multicultural surroundings. They measure intellectual capital (knowledge of global issues, networks, organizations, strategies, and so on), psychological capital (strong psychological attributes, openness, curiosity, cosmopolitanism, and so on), and social capital (ability to work with others and build relationships and networks in multicultural settings) (Javidan et al., 2007).

A globalist approach to culture asserts the need for an integrated understanding of not only the facts about cultural groups but the social and psychological capabilities of adapting and adjusting to rapidly changing cultural identities and formations (Huntington, 1997). History provides us with many examples of the battles between cultures. However, the technologies and understandings about social gaps and conflict are more advanced than they use to be in ways that enhance general understanding about social and political behavior. The cultural splits and groupings "animated by religion and politics" will require a more complex "understanding of culture, not new technology or science" (Ikle, 2006). In short, they will require a deeper understanding of the "software of the mind."

Determination of Intent

IC and national-security analysts have long been interested in determining intent and motivation with cultural accuracy. There is an increasing need to understand "hearts and minds" at a strategic level because of the effect they can have, for example, in exacerbating an insurgency in Iraq. Cultural ignorance at an operational level can lead to negative public opinion and at a tactical level can endanger both civilians and troops. A lack of continued research and training regarding adversaries' cultures can have grave consequences strategically, operationally, and tactically (McFate, 2005; Freakley, 2005).

Efforts to enhance cultural awareness and to determine the intentions of political adversaries and supporters are not new. Cultural training in the U.S. military began during the Indian Wars of 1865-1885 and resulted in the Bureau of American Ethnology. During World War II, anthropologists served the war effort directly, first conducting intelligence operations in Burma for the Office of Strategic Services and later advising on how to generate political stability in target countries through a process known as schizmogenesis. American anthropologists produced studies, for example, that by ethnographer Ruth Benedict (1946), *The Chrysanthemum and the Sword*, which concerned the Japanese national character.

Understanding one's friends and enemies requires not only intelligence from a satellite photo of an arms dump but intelligence about a group's cultural interests, habits, intentions, beliefs, social organizations, and political symbols. New adversaries and operational environments necessitate a sharper focus on cultural knowledge of not only adversaries but also supporters to avoid grave consequences. Understanding the culture of an adversary can make a positive difference strategically, operationally, and tactically (McFate, 2005; Kipp et al., 2006).

Although future success in "reading minds and intentions" will depend on cultural knowledge, DOD lacks the programs, systems, models, personnel, and organizations to deal with either an existing threat or the changing cultural environment. At a strategic level, understanding "minds" in Iraq will require a better understanding of the tribal nature of the Iraqi culture and society and of why power struggles have reverted to the tribe. Once Sunnis were humiliated in the conflict and frozen out of their jobs through the disbanding of the Iraqi military or de-Baathification, the tribal network became the backbone of the insurgency as a direct result of U.S. misunderstanding of the Iraqi culture (McFate, 2005). Understanding local culture and mindset can make a favorable difference strategically, operationally, and tactically. More broadly, "reading the Arab mind" requires attention to a regional and collective mindset with respect to values about child-rearing, evaluation of male-female relationships, and boy-girl differences (Patai and De Atkine, 2007).

A current initiative addressing "anthropology and a level of knowledge concerning a wide range of culture" is the U.S. Army's Human Terrain System (HTS). The core building block of the system is a five-person human terrain team (HTT) that will be embedded in each forward-deployed brigade or regimental staff. The HTT will provide a commander with experienced officers, civilians, and social scientists who are trained and skilled in cultural research and analysis. Current intelligence systems and organizations remain traditionally structured and collect battlefield elements of information to support commanders in physical combat. As contemporary conflicts have moved further from combat involving regular formations and heavy maneuvering warfare, it has become apparent that technical battle information has diminished in importance relative to the requirements for ethnographic, economic, and cultural information to stabilize an indigenous government (Kipp et al., 2006; Packer, 2007; Kilcullen, 2007).

What is the future of the understanding and evaluation of human intent? What are the implications for national security? To begin with, any theories that advance the ability to determine intent in the context of multicultural interactions will continue to put forth that cultural behaviors and psychological patterns are interrelated. Sociocultural and psychological models will advance a deeper understanding of psychological processes in a cultural context (Asch, 1953; Bruner, 1990; Hastorf and Cantril, 1954).

There will be a trend for advances in cross-cultural understanding of intention and meaning to occur in a cross-cultural comparative research. For example, traditional social-science models built primarily on Western assumptions will be challenged. In particular, a bias that is invisible to many psychological and social-science models assumes that Western social-science models regarding what is normal are universal. Therefore, cross-cultural comparative research can be pursued to validate or invalidate many of the European and American psychological models that assume that basic processes of brain function and human behavior are universal.

Traditional social-choice research concludes that individualism that prevails in European American models of psychology predicts individuality and preferences for freedom and control (Markus, 2007). That is illustrated in the cultural-orientations assessments and profiles of European Americans who tend to prefer environmental control, equality as a power value, and individualism as a core value (Price, 2007). There is an assumption in Western models of choice that those who choose for themselves are happier, are healthier, and perform better than those who do not get to choose (Brehm, 1956; Deci and Ryan, 1987). However, having more choice or decision options is not necessarily preferred. A disjointed (individualism-independent) or conjointed (collectivism-interdependent) psychological construct of the self in choice-making is determined by whether the cultural patterns are Western or Eastern, respectively (Markus, 2007). That can have implications for the processes of Western ideals of freedom and democracy.

Research will continue to determine the effects of culture on the brain. To date, this research has taken two routes: studies of neuroplasticity that provide insight into the effects of social experience on the brain and studies of brain evolution that provide insight into natural selection and the brain. Cultural change and acculturation are evident in studies, for example, of the "reorganization of the brain" (neuroplasticity) in response to adaptation. Future research may also advance undertanding of cross-cultural differences in object-processing regions of the brain (Chen, 2007).

Measurement of brain activity of Western and Chinese people has provided neuroimaging evidence that culture shapes how the self is represented in the human brain (Zhu et al., 2007). When judging self-relevant items, both Western and Chinese participants showed activation in the medial prefrontal cortex (MPFC). Further research may lead to better understanding of the neural basis of cultural differences in fundamental processes of cognition, emotion, and motivation. That would be an important future direction, although logistical hurdles would need to be dealt with for this field to thrive (for example, comparing functional magnetic-resonance images between groups presents problems of reliability and requires that studies be done in the same location). Other research on cultural dimensions includes the work done by Aycan et al. (2000) on cultural fatalism, by Gelfand et al. (2006) on the construct of cultural tightness-looseness (strength of social norms), by Bond et al. (2004) on social axioms (cynicism, spirituality, and reward for allocation), and by Shalom Schwartz (1994) on values at the individual and cultural levels.

Research will advance understanding of systematic cross-cultural differences in the anatomical structure and function of the brain. Many of the variations in brain functions appear to be rooted in culture-dependent experiences, such as language experience and early learning, as well as by variations in neuronal genes. Future research will probably examine gene-culture interactions as a way to understand historical adaptation by social groups (Chen, 2007).

Dan Sperber, a cognitive anthropologist, proposes that research on culture be understood as an epidemiology of mental representations; this would translate to the spread of ideas and practices from person to person.[2] The mathematical tools of epidemiology (how diseases spread) and of population biology (how genes and organisms spread) can be used to understand cultural evolution (Pinker, 2002). Research in neurolinguistic programming (NLP) as an interpersonal approach will also advance the subjective study of language, communication, and personal change in a cross-cultural context (Laborde, 1984; Moine and Lloyd, 2007).[3]

The application of NLP to negotiation, sales, and communication has not been validated in a cross-cultural context. Generally, NLP aims to increase behavioral flexibility (choice) by understanding how a person thinks about a problem or a desired outcome. Rather than just listening to and responding to someone, NLP aims to respond to nonverbal communication, such as tone, gesture, posture, and eye movements. Nonverbal cues reveal information not typically available when one is distracted by preconceptions or expectations. Research on NLP methods and questioning is intended to clarify what has been left out or distorted in verbal communication. These approaches are used to reframe thinking and to become aware of others' preferences for communication that might not be one's own. The greatest challenge in current cross-cultural communication research is the difficulty in reading others' minds when one's own mind has cultural filters and biases about values and intentions.

It is important to note that there is also increased research interest in how meditation, empathy, compassion, and suffering are represented in the brain. William Mobley, of Stanford University, argues that these traditionally are subjects that "neuroscientists avoid . . . because we don't understand them" (Baker, 2005). Last, the field of neuroeconomics is another recent research agenda that uses neuroscience methods to understand cooperation, decision making, fairness, among others (Sanfey et al., 2003; Zak, 2004; Loewenstein et al., 2008) This field may also be integrated with cross-cultural theory and methods.

Finding and Recommendation

Finding 4-1. There is a growing awareness in the U.S. government that effective engagement in a complex world—commercially, militarily, and diplomatically—will increasingly require an unbiased understanding of foreign cultures. Research

---

[2]See Sperber's biography online at http://en.wikipedia.org/wiki/Dan_Sperber. Last accessed on June 23, 2008.

[3]Neurolinguistic programming is defined as the study of the human subjective experience and of how it provides a structure for all behavior. Neurolinguistic programming was created specifically to understand how verbal communication and nonverbal communication affect the human brain and enhance management of otherwise automatic neurological functions.

is enhancing understanding of how culture affects human cognition, including brain functioning, and is even suggesting a link between culture and brain development. The U.S. military is placing greater emphasis on cultural-awareness training and education as a critical element in its strategy for engaging in current and future conflicts. Military conflicts will increasingly involve prolonged interaction with civilian populations in which cultural awareness will be a matter of life and death and a major factor in outcomes. Similarly, political leaders, diplomats, intelligence officers, corporate executives, and academicians will need a deeper, more sophisticated understanding of foreign cultures to communicate more effectively with their counterparts in non-Western societies in the era of globalization.

Recommendation 4-1. The growing U.S. government interest in cultural training and education is well placed, and its investment in related research and development and in practical training should be substantially increased. Training programs, to be most effective, should be developed and implemented on a multidisciplinary basis. Investment should be made particularly in neuroscience research on the effects of culture on human cognition, with special attention to the relationship between culture and brain development.

ETHICAL IMPLICATIONS OF COGNITIVE NEUROSCIENCE AND RELATED TECHNOLOGIES

Introduction

Modern bioethics is a complex field that emerged in the late 1960s among a small group of philosophers, theologians, and physicians.[4] Motivated by such dramatic developments in the life sciences as the decoding of deoxyribonucleic acid (DNA), experiments in organ transplantation, the introduction of renal dialysis, and advances in end-of-life interventions, those thinkers found ethical traditions to be stressed in addressing novel moral questions. The Hippocratic oath emphasized the avoidance of intentionally harming patients, maintaining confidentiality, and respecting fraternal and guild-like professional relationships but was silent about telling patients the truth or obtaining their informed consent. Nor did traditional medical ethics address balancing individual and group interests or society's role in providing access to health care.

External factors also played an important role in stimulating the early development of bioethics. The patients'-rights movement emerged as a variant of other civil-rights movements, especially for psychiatric patients and their advocates. Treatment of stigmatized diseases, such as cancer, began to show signs of

---

[4]The "small group" referred to was in the United States and led to the creation of the first two bioethics research centers, The Hastings Center (1969) and the Kennedy Institute of Ethics at Georgetown University (1971).

improvement and to stimulate a demand for more information and control for patients and a greater interest in communication in the doctor-patient relationship. And litigation became a more prevalent method of resolving disputes.

Medical schools gradually introduced more systematic ethics education into their curricula and appointed professors of medical ethics. The term *bioethics* became popular because it suggested consideration of ethical issues in the life sciences generally, not only in clinical medicine. During the middle 1970s, problems of consent to medical treatment of those who could not speak for themselves sparked a national debate, and ethics committees were instituted in hospitals partly to clarify the values at stake in difficult cases and partly to settle disagreements among caregivers and family members without resort to the courts.

Two important characteristics of bioethics are the large and continuing role of scandals in the growth of the field and the prominence of public commissions in the development of its canon and in advancing its social legitimacy. A 1966 paper in the *New England Journal of Medicine* by a distinguished Harvard professor of anesthesiology asserted that ethical problems in human research trials were rampant and cited nearly two dozen published papers in which examples of unethical conduct were claimed to be evident (Beecher, 1966a,b). Social-science studies, such as Stanley Milgram's "obedience to authority" experiment, also called attention to professional ethics (Milgram, 1973, 1974).

No incident so rocked the medical world as the 1972 revelation of the U.S. Public Health Service syphilis study in which 400 black men who had tertiary syphilis were observed for 40 years without consent and without penicillin therapy when it became available (Moreno, 2001). Among the public responses to the syphilis-study scandal was the formation of the National Commission for the Protection of Human Subjects of Biomedical and Behavioral Research (1974-1978).[5] The commission proposed specific protections for particular populations that it identified as vulnerable—including children, pregnant women, and prisoners—and informed consent and prior review of experiment proposals by a special committee, the latter conditions to apply to all research subjects. With some modifications, those proposals were codified and continue to be the basis of the U.S. research protection system to this day. All federal agencies that fund or sponsor human-subjects research are supposed to be in compliance with the "common rule," and several agencies have more specific regulations, depending on their missions. Any institution or organization that receives federal research funds and any entity that volunteers to be in compliance regardless of the funding source are also covered by the common rule. A few states have instituted regulations governing particular forms of research. Current guidelines for ethical recruitment and participation of human volunteers in research generally prohibit participation by prisoners, due to actual or potential coercion risk. There is a

---

[5]The National Commission for the Protection of Human Subjects of Biomedical and Behavioral Research was established under Title II of Public Law 93-348, Section 201(a).

general challenge in conducting research that might actually be aimed at helping the prisoners to regain function or improve certain functions, and whether they are able to give informed consent (IOM, 2006). More recent and related commissions include the President's Commission on Ethical Problems in Medicine and Biomedical and Behavioral Research (1980-1984), the National Bioethics Advisory Commission (1996-2000), and the President's Council on Bioethics (2001-present).

There are several sanctions for failure to comply with research regulations. The federal Office for Human Research Protections may find that an institution has failed to comply with the relevant regulations and therefore halt current protocols. The Food and Drug Administration (FDA) may find that drug or device development has failed to comply with the regulations and withhold licensure for marketing. Investigators may lose their sponsor's financial support and be subjected to limitations of their ability to conduct future clinical trials. Editors of professional journals may refuse to publish papers that include "tainted" data or, if the data are sound in spite of demonstrated ethical lapses, publish only with specific attention to those failings. In some instances, litigation may ensue, especially if failure to comply is associated with an injury in the course of research.

Recently, investigators' and sponsors' financial conflicts of interest have become a matter of general concern. There is evidence that study design and timely release of data have been influenced by proprietary considerations. Conversely, decisions about which promising lines of research are pursued are surely influenced by market concerns, especially as government support of science declines. Those problems, too, have been brought into the ambit of bioethics.

On the whole, however, the system of protections for human research subjects is not well designed to capture instances of intentional wrongdoing. Rather, it provides guidance for well-motivated investigators who wish to be in compliance with regulatory requirements and practice standards. In part, that limitation results from the system's being based on paper reporting rather than in situ audits of professional conduct. Yet the scrutiny associated with the prevailing system does seem to provide some check on individual investigator discretion.

In contrast with bioethical principles that are well established, such as the obligation to obtain the informed consent of competent subjects, there are many unresolved questions. For example, under what circumstances is a deceptive research design, as is common in social psychology, ethically acceptable? When is it justifiable to involve persons in research whose decision-making capacity is diminished, such as persons with neurological disorders? Those sorts of problems continue to excite a great deal of debate in science and ethics.

Professionals in the life sciences and many laypersons are generally aware of the history and requirements of human-subjects research in the civilian world, but far fewer appreciate the long and complex history of such considerations in the military and in the IC. In fact, human-experiments policies in the national-security world preceded, and to some extent anticipated, policies that were created only much later in the world of civilian biomedicine. A striking example is the appearance of the first consent form in a medical experiment, which was probably devised by U.S. Army Major Walter Reed in the course of his yellow fever experiments in Cuba in 1900. Reed's brilliant and arduous efforts and those of his colleagues (one of whom died as the result of exposure to the bite of a carrier mosquito) not only led to the virtual elimination of a fearful scourge but exemplified an advance in the treatment of experiment volunteers—in this case, soldiers and Spanish immigrant laborers (Moreno, 2001). (It must be said, however, that both the circumstances of recruitment of the laborers and the financial inducement offered would probably not be acceptable today.)

Nearly 50 years later, 23 Nazi doctors and bureaucrats were tried at Nuremberg for crimes involving horrific experiments on concentration-camp inmates. The experiments listed in the indictment included several that were sponsored by the Luftwaffe, such as studies of explosive decompression and hypothermia. Both were tied to unanswered clinical questions of interest to the medical corps. The defendants appealed to the doctrine of superior orders and to a utilitarian justification that many lives could be saved by jeopardizing the lives of a few people already slated for death. They further noted that the allied governments had themselves engaged in human experiments on captive populations for national-security purposes during the war, such as a malaria study involving 800 federal prisoners. The three American judges finally rejected the defense arguments and sentenced eight of the defendants to death and eight others to long prison terms for complicity in murder, but they were sufficiently impressed by the apparent absence of international experiment standards that they decided to write their own (Moreno, 2001). The third part of the tribunal's decision is known as the Nuremberg Code. The first sentence is famous and reads, "The voluntary consent of the human subject is absolutely essential." A number of other principles that were articulated would elicit wide agreement today but were not necessarily well established at the time, such as the right of the volunteer to leave an experiment at any time.[6]

It is remarkable that the national-security–related interest in human-experiment rules was unfolding in the United States at precisely the same time as the Nuremburg Tribunals, but not in public. Early in 1947, the new Atomic Energy Commission discovered that its predecessor, the Manhattan Engineer District (better known as the Manhattan Project), had sponsored the injection of plutonium into 17 hospitalized patients, apparently as part of an effort to establish the human excretion rate for the sake of young laboratory workers who might be exposed to the newly isolated metal. The commission decided not to release information about those sensitive experiments to the public, but it determined that

---

[6]Nuremberg Military Tribunals. 1949. Trials of War Criminals before the Nuremberg Military Tribunals under Control Council Law. No. 10, Vol. 2, pp. 181-182. Washington, D.C.: U.S. Government Printing Office. Available from http://ohsr.od.nih.gov/guidelines/nuremberg.html. Last accessed June 18, 2008.

its contractors to whom it released radioisotopes for medical studies would have to obtain the subjects' "informed consent." That was the first time that phrase appeared, as far as is known. However, the requirement seems to have been at best poorly applied and to have disappeared from institutional memory by the early 1950s (Moreno, 2001).

As the early Cold War era unfolded, DOD contemplated the need to engage in human experiments involving atomic, biological, and chemical agents for defensive purposes. In a secret consultation process, several DOD advisory committees were asked to develop recommendations for the conduct of such experiments. Finally, the department's general counsel proposed that the Nuremberg Code, penned by three American judges only a few years before, apply to the atomic, biological, and chemical "(ABC) warfare" experiments to avoid the U.S. hypocrisy of not following the code. Secretary Charles M. Wilson adopted the proposal shortly after taking office in 1953 but included a written consent requirement. That caused consternation among the advisory committees that seem largely to have opposed the adoption of any such formal policy, considering it an unnecessary departure from prior practices and a dangerous precedent that could undermine military and medical authority (Wilson, 1953).

The Wilson policy made little difference in the conduct of national-security-related scientific and technological exercises. Perhaps the most graphic example of the failure of the policy was the deployment of over 200,000 soldiers and marines within a few miles of ground zero at atomic test shots throughout the 1950s. Those deployments were regarded as training exercises rather than as medical experiments. In contrast, the Army lysergic acid diethylamide (LSD) experiments of the 1960s were accompanied by some informed-consent processes, however minimal and inadequate. By 1975, the Army inspector general concluded that the Wilson policy had failed. Interestingly, some of the wording of the original memo has survived in current military regulations on human experimentation, such as Army Regulation 70-25 (Moreno, 2001).

Those examples raise the question of policy-makers' attitudes toward the use of military personnel in medical experiments. On the whole, the attitude of both World War II and Cold War–era authorities seems to have been that, although the risks associated with a medical experiment in military service might pale in comparison with those encountered in combat, it seemed important not to reduce young men and women in uniform to the status of human guinea pigs. Thus, alternative populations were often sought, including in at least some cases hospitalized psychiatric patients. In the last few years, however, new information has emerged concerning the exposure of sailors and soldiers to active nerve agents during the 1960s.

Secret military and intelligence-related human experiments seem to have ceased after the Army and CIA scandals of the middle 1970s, and a vastly more sensitive attitude on these matters appears to have prevailed, although some insist that secret experiments should continue, citing the development of the anthrax vaccine as an example. What seems to be unassailable is that military authorities are loath to violate informed-consent standards without justification (in accordance with the Uniform Code of Military Justice) or without authorization by appropriate civilian authorities.[7] Thus, DOD sought and received from FDA a waiver of informed consent for the voluntary use of some compounds during the first Gulf War. Although the waiver was controversial, especially after the war, that it was sought is noteworthy. The stated motive for the waiver request was the concern that military personnel could be exposed to agents (such as nerve gas and botulinum toxin) for which there was no approved therapy but substantial evidence in other contexts that the compounds in question could be protective. Under the Uniform Code of Military Justice, members of the armed forces are required to obey all lawful orders, including those involving medical care that may maintain or re-establish their ability to do their job. However, they are under no obligation to participate in a medical experiment.

Today, the formal procedures in place for the use of military personnel in medical experiments are at least as stringent—and probably far more stringent—than those common in industry and academe. That implies not that no abuses can occur, nor that convenient alternative frameworks (such as field testing) cannot be used to circumvent the research rules, but only that the official policies and procedures in the military are rigorous.

The IC is subject to the same common provisions of informed consent and prior review although it is claimed that no human experiments are performed by intelligence agencies. An interesting and unresolved policy dilemma is whether classified research can ever be ethically sound inasmuch as it lacks transparency, such as in the form of public accountability. For example, if a member of an ethics review board disagrees with a majority decision involving a classified human experiment, that member would be unable to engage in a public protest of that decision.

A contemporary problem is the status of detainees at military installations who are suspects in the war on terrorism.[8] Presumably, the ethical standards that apply to all human research subjects should apply to them as well. But if they are not protected by the provisions of the Geneva protocols for prisoners of war, the question would be whether as potential research subjects they are nonetheless

---

[7]The Uniform Code of Military Justice is available from http://www4.law.cornell.edu/uscode/10/stApIIch47.html. Last accessed March 27, 2008.

[8]Acts of terrorism do not in themselves imply that the perpetrators have a fundamentally different neurological constitution from other human beings. Our own social and political history is rife with examples of behavior that terrorized those who felt themselves to be potential targets—guerilla actions during the Revolution and the Civil War, racist lynchings, labor insurrections, domestic rebel movements, and presidential assassinations. Often, the perpetrators have been called radicals or anarchists rather than terrorists, but the principle is the same. Like today's foreign terrorists, some may be attracted for many reasons to an extremist ideology, including an exceptionally rigid idealism, youthful immaturity, physical or psychological coercion, psychopathological conditions, or some combination of them. Such conditions are not peculiar to an ethnic, national, racial, or religious group.

protected by other international conventions, such as the Universal Declaration of Human Rights (United Nations, 1948). Those technical questions of international law are beyond the scope of this report.

One striking conclusion to be drawn from this brief history is that, as far as is known, no U.S. administration has ever declared that the human-experiment rules could be suspended because of a national emergency. That cannot be said of Nazi Germany: the Third Reich ignored an Interior Ministry guidance from 1931 that was still technically in effect. Nor did the imperial Japanese government hesitate to engage in human experiments with biological and chemical weapons in Manchuria that rivaled or even exceeded the Nazi experiments in barbarity.

Less is known about America's traditional allies, which have been far less candid about their research activities on sensitive issues. One interesting recent exception is the sarin gas experiments at Porton Down in the United Kingdom during the 1950s. Revelations associated with the 1953 death of a British soldier in one of those experiments led to a new inquest in 2005 that cast some light on the work and raised grave questions about the consent and safety procedures in place at the time.[9]

Ethics, Cognitive Neuroscience, and National-Security Research

The field of bioethics has spawned several related fields—clinical ethics, research ethics, and public-health ethics—and more recently has given rise to neuroethics.[10] Intensive interest in the ethical issues raised by the rapid advances in neuroscience led first to several academic conferences in the early 2000s, then to a spate of literature, and now to the creation of a professional organization and at least two academic journals. Among the topics addressed in neuroethics are the nature of personal identity, human dignity, and autonomy in light of various novel surgical and pharmacological interventions; the relationship between mind and body in light of new information about brain processes; the implications of neural imaging for privacy; neurogenetics and behavior control; and the management of suspicious results of neuroimaging research.

Discussions of neuroethics and human experiments for national-security purposes generate concerns that go beyond the already controversial topics of human experiments and national security.[11] Because the modern world views the brain as the organ most closely associated with personal identity and modern

---

[9]For additional information on neuroethics and the law, please see http://www.press.uchicago. edu/cgi-bin/hfs.cgi/00/16495.ctl. The American Association for the Advancement of Science has a related program that may be viewed online at http://www.aaas.org/spp/sfrl/projects/neuroscience/. Last accessed on June 19, 2008.

[10]Neuroethics is a phenomenon mainly in the English-speaking world, including the United States, Canada, the United Kingdom, and Australia. However, interest in Europe appears to be growing, to judge by personal communications of the committee.

[11]The topic of the nature of research necessary to prepare American military forces to withstand various kinds of potential behavior-modifying techniques is not addressed in this report.

democratic theory values the individual as a rights-bearer and moral agent, there is sure to be enormous societal interest in any prospective manipulation of neural processes. American society experienced a telling episode along those lines during the 1950s, when "brain-washing" became part of popular culture—and IC experiments—after the treasonous statements of American prisoners of war in captivity in North Korea. Although anxieties about clandestine U.S. government activities are easy to deride, later Army and CIA experiments involving hallucinogens were associated with at least two deaths in 1953 and with multiple exposures of ordinary citizens.

Serious contemporary ethical discussion of neuroscience and national-security policy carries an unusual historical burden. The current underlying science and resulting technology are far more sophisticated and, to many, threatening to personal autonomy and human dignity. Proponents of the science may well argue that neuroscience promises to enhance rather than undermine dignity and autonomous choice, but that point of view is not always the prevalent one, especially when national-security goals are viewed with suspicion. Examples of neuroscience experiments that may have implications for national security are numerous. Virtually all involve what has been called "dual use" research applicable to military, intelligence, or policing, as well as health-care, purposes.

International Standards and Controls

Research with human subjects is guided by several international documents that are discussed in detail in Appendix E; there are also numerous international harmonization initiatives that apply to drug development and regulation and to environmental risk assessment and management. In Europe, research is further governed by the European Medicines Agency (EMEA)[12] and the European Forum for Good Clinical Practice (EFGCP).[13] As discussed previously in this report, in the United States, FDA and the Department of Health and Human Services Common Rule (45 CFR 46) guide drug and device development and human-subjects research in general (United States Department of Health and Human Services, 2005). Nations other than the United States and the European Union may have their own specific rules and directives, but not much is known about the extent to which they are implemented and complied with.

It should be noted that the United States is not necessarily in a position of moral superiority to other countries with regard to practices; as noted above, there are serious questions about the extent to which the research house in the United States is in order. Nonetheless, it can be said at least that the developed world

---

[12]For additional information, see EMEA's Web site, http://www.emea.europa.eu/. Last accessed on December 20, 2007.

[13]For additional information, see EFGCP's Web site, http::://www.efgcp.org. Last accessed on December 20, 2007.

has established fairly well-articulated ethical standards and that there are various avenues for addressing egregious violations.

However, several questions remain about the adequacy of the protection of human beings as subjects of biomedical research related to cognitive neuroscience, especially in confidential or military contexts. For example, How great is the impact of international ethical rules and regulations governing human-subjects research, such as the Declaration of Helsinki (DoH) (World Medical Association, 1964)? The DoH is essentially an internationally accepted document, but some countries might not comply with it. How are international rules and standards respected by individual countries? How is compliance enforced? How much overlap is there between national and international requirements for the protection of subjects of research involving human beings?

REFERENCES

Published

Aperian Global. 2007. GLOBESMART COMMANDER and GLOBESMART SOLDIER: Helping Remove the Fog of War. Aperian Press Release. San Francisco, CA, April 9, 2007. Available from http://www.aperianglobal.com/about_aperian_global_news.asp. Last accessed March 26, 2008.

Asch, S.E. 1953. Effects of group pressure upon the modification and distortion of judgements. Pp. 151-162 in *Group Dynamics: Research and Theory.* D. Cartwright, and A. Zander, eds. Evanston, IL: Row Peterson.

Aycan, Z., R.N. Kanungo, M. Mendonca, K. Yu, J. Deller, G. Stahl, and A. Kurshid. 2000. Impact of culture on human resource management practices: A 10-country comparison. *Applied Psychology: An International Review* 49(1):192-220.

Baker, Mitzi. 2005. Dalai Lama and neuroscientists build bridge between Buddhism and Western medicine. Press release. Stanford University. Available from http://med.stanford.edu/events/dalailama/full_story.html. Last accessed March 26, 2008.

Beecher, Henry K. 1966a. Consent in clinical experimentation: Myth and reality. *Journal of the American Medical Association* 195:34-35.

Beecher, Henry K. 1966b. Ethics and clinical research. *New England Journal of Medicine* 274:1354-1360.

Benedict, Ruth. 1946. *The Chrysanthemum and the Sword.* Boston, MA: Houghton, Mifflin Company.

Bond, M.H., K. Leung, A. Au, K-K Tong, S.R. Carrasquel, F. Murakami, S. Yamaguchi, G. Bierbrauer, T.M. Singelis, M. Broer, F. Boen, S.M. Lambert, M.C. Ferreira, K.A. Noels, J. Bavel, S. Safdar, J. Zhang, L. Chen, I. Solcova, I. Stetovska, T. Niit, K-K. Niit, H. Hurme, M. Böling, V. Franchi, G. Magradze, N. Javakhishvili, K. Boehnke, E. Klinger, X. Huang, M. Fulop, M. Berkics, P. Panagiotopoulou, S. Sriram, N. Chaudhary, A. Ghosh, N. Vohra, D.F. Iqbal, J. Kurman, R.D. Thein, A.L. Comunian, K.A. Son, I. Austers, C. Harb, J.O.T. Odusanya, Z.A. Ahmed, R. Ismail, F. Vijver, C. Ward, A. Mogaji, D.L. Sam, M.J.Z. Khan, W.E. Cabanillas, L. Sycip, F. Neto, R. Cabecinhas, P. Xavier, M. Dinca, N. Lebedeva, A. Viskochil, O. Ponomareva, S.M. Burgess, L. Oceja, S. Campo, K-K. Hwang, J.B. D'souza, B. Ataca, A. Furnham, and I.R. Lewis. 2004. Culture-level dimensions of social axioms and their correlates across 41 cultures. *Journal of Cross-Cultural Psychology* 35(5):548-570.

Brehm, J.W. 1956. Postdecision changes in the desirability of alternatives. *Journal of Abnormal and Social Psychology* 52(3):384-389.

Bruner, J.S. 1990. *Acts of Meaning*. Cambridge, MA: Harvard University Press.

Dahl, Stephan. 2000. *Intercultural Skills for Business*. London, UK: ECE.

Deci, E.L., and R.M. Ryan. 1987. The support of autonomy and the control of behavior. *Journal of Personality and Social Psychology* 53(6):1024-1037.

Freakley, Benjamin C. 2005. Cultural awareness and combat power. *Infantry Magazine* 94(March-April):1-2.

Friedman, Thomas L. 2005. *The World Is Flat: A Brief History of the Twenty First Century*. New York, NY: Farrar, Straus and Giroux.

Gelfand, Michele J., Lisa H. Nishii, and Jana L. Raver. 2006. On the nature and importance of cultural tightness-looseness. *Journal of Applied Psychology* 91(6):1225-1244.

Harris, Phillip R., Robert T. Moran, and Sarah V. Moran. 2004. *Managing Cultural Differences: Global Leadership Strategies for the Twenty First Century*. Oxford, UK: Elsevier Butterworth-Heinemann.

Hastorf, A., and H. Cantril. 1954. They saw a game: A case study. *Journal of Abnormal and Social Psychology* 49:129-134

Huntington, Samuel. 1997. *The Clash of Civilizations and Remaking of World Order*. New York, NY: Simon and Schuster.

Ikle, Fred Charles. 2006. *Annihilation from Within: The Ultimate Threat to Nations*. New York, NY: Columbia University Press.

IOM (Institute of Medicine). 2006. *Ethical Considerations for Research Involving Prisoners*. Washington, D.C.: The National Academies Press. Available from http://www.iom.edu/CMS/3740/24594/35792.aspx. Last accessed on June 20, 2008.

Javidan, Mansour, Richard M. Steers, and Michael A. Hitt. 2007. *The Global Mindset (Advances in International Management)*. Oxford, UK: Elsevier/Jai Press.

Kilcullen, David J. 2007. Understanding current operations in Iraq. *Small Wars Journal*. Available from http://smallwarsjournal.com/blog/2007/06/understanding-current-operatio/. Last accessed March 27, 2008.

Kipp, Jacob, Lester Grau, Karl Prinslow, and Don Smith. 2006. The Human Terrain System: A CORDS for the 21st century. *Military Review* 86 (September-October 2006):8-15. Available from http://usacac.leavenworth.army.mil/CAC/milreview/English/sepoct06/kipp.pdf. Last Accessed February 11, 2008.

Laborde, Genie Z. 1984. *Influencing with Integrity: Management Skills for Communication and Negotiation*. Palo Alto, CA: Syntony Publishing.

Loewenstein, George, Scott Rick, and Jonathan D. Cohen. 2008. Neuroeconomics. *Annual Review of Psychology* 59 (January):647-672.

McFate, Montgomery. 2005. The military utility of understanding adversary culture. *Joint Force Quarterly* 38:42-48.

Milgram, Stanley. 1973. The perils of obedience. *Harper's Magazine,* December.

Milgram, Stanley. 1974. *Obedience to Authority: An Experimental View*. New York, NY: Harper and Row.

Moine, Donald, and Ken Lloyd. 2007. *Ultimate Selling Power*. Franklin Lakes, NJ: Career Press.

Moreno, Jonathan D. 2001. *Undue Risk: Secret State Experiments on Humans*. New York, NY: Routledge.

NRC (National Research Council). 2008. *Human Behavior in Military Contexts*. Washington, DC: The National Academies Press. Available from http://www.nap.edu/catalog.php?record_id=12023.

Packer, George. 2007. A report at large: Knowing the enemy. *The New Yorker*, November 28. Available from http://www.newyorker.com/archive/2006/12/18/06121fa_fact2?currentPage=2. Last accessed June 18, 2008.

Patai, Raphael, and Norvell B. De Atkine. 2007. *The Arab Mind*. New York, NY: Hatherleigh Press.

Pinker, Steven. 2002. *The Black Slate: The Modern Denial of Human Nature*. New York, NY: Penguin Books.

Rudd, Jill E., and Diana R. Lawson. 2007. *Communicating in Global Business Negotiations: A Geocentric Approach*. Thousand Oaks, CA: Sage Publications.

Sanfey, A.G., J.K. Rilling, J.A. Aronson, L.E. Nystrom, and J.D. Cohen. 2003. The neural basis of economic decision-making in the ultimatum game. *Science* 300(5626):1755-1758.

Schmitz, Joerg. 2005. *Cultural Orientation Guide: The Roadmap to Cultural Competence*. Princeton, NJ: Princeton Training Press.

Schwartz, Shalom H. 1994. Are there universal aspects in the structure and contents of human values? *Journal of Social Issues* 50(4):19-45.

Thomas, David C., and Kerr Inkson. 2004. *Cultural Intelligence: People Skills for Global Business*. San Francisco, CA: Berret-Koehler.

Trompenaars, Alfons, and Charles Hampden-Turner. 1998. *Riding the Waves of Culture*. New York, NY: McGraw Hill.

United Nations. 1948. Universal Declaration of Human Rights. Adopted and proclaimed by General Assembly Resolution 217 A (III) of December 10, 1948. Palais de Chaillot, Paris, December 1948. Available from http://www.un.org/Overview/rights.html.

United States Department of Health and Human Services. 2005. Code of Federal Regulations. 45 CFR 46. Protection of Human Subjects. Washington, DC, June. Available from http://www.hhs. gov/ohrp/humansubjects/guidance/45cfr46.htm. Last accessed June 18, 2008.

Viotti, Paul R., and Mark V. Kauppi. 1987. *International Relations Theory: Realism, Pluralism, Globalism*. New York, NY: Macmillan.

Walker, Danielle, Thomas Walker, and Joerg Schmitz. 2003. *Doing Business Internationally: The Guide to Cross-Cultural Success,* 2nd Edition. New York, NY: McGraw-Hill.

Wilson, C.E. 1953. Memorandum from Secretary of Defense C.E. Wilson to Secretary of the Army, Secretary of the Navy, Secretary of the Air Force. Subject: "Use of Human Volunteers in Experimental Research," February 26, 1953. Available from http://www.gwu.edu/~nsarchiv/radiation/ dir/mstreet/commeet/meet2/brief2/tab_i/br2i1b.txt. Last accessed June 18, 2008.

World Medical Association. 1964. Declaration of Helsinki: Ethical Principles for Medical Research Involving Human Subjects. Adopted by the 18th World Medical Association General Assembly. Helsinki, Finland, June 1964. Available from http://www.wma.net/e/policy/b3.htm. Last accessed June 18, 2008.

Zak, Paul J. 2004. Neuroeconomics. *Philosophical Transactions of the Royal Society Biology* 359(1451):1737-1748.

Zhu, Ying, Jin Fan Li Zhang, and Shihui Han. 2007. Neural basis of cultural influence on self-representation. *NeuroImage* 34(3):1310-1316.

Unpublished

Chen, Chuansheng. 2007. "Culture, Brain, and Cognition: A Few Comments." Presentation to the committee on October 31, 2007.

Markus, Hazel. 2007. "Culture Matters." Presentation to the committee on October 31, 2007.

Price, Kenneth. 2007. "Defining and Applying Cultural Anthropology." Presentation to the committee on October 31, 2007.

5

Potential Intelligence and Military Applications of Cognitive Neuroscience and Related Technologies

INTRODUCTION

Chapter 2 discusses the basis of neuroscience and neurotechnologies, and Chapter 3 describes apparent trends in neuroscience and neurotechnologies. This chapter applies the technology-warning method developed in *Avoiding Surprise in an Era of Global Technology Advances* (NRC, 2005) to particular fields of science and technology that potentially have important military applications. In some cases, the committee amplifies the technology-warning method to illustrate how neurophysiological research and cognitive and neural research conducted in other countries might affect assessments.

Appendix C (Chapter 2 from *Avoiding Surprise*) sets forth in great detail the background and purpose of the technology-warning method and defines the key terms listed in technology-assessment Charts 5-1 through 5-8 below in this chapter. Readers will find it helpful to read Appendix C before reading this chapter. In keeping with the main subjects of interest identified in Chapter 2, the examples below are meant to be representational depictions of future military applications. Figure 5-1 illustrates cross-functional information flow and outlines one possible solution to analyzing cognitive neuroscience research by intelligence analysts.

At the base of Figure 5-1 are examples of sources and types of information that must be collected. Sources of neuroscience information should include the public sector, the private sector, and the intelligence community. That information needs to be analyzed and applied to the technology-warning methodology. Afterward, the information will need to be analyzed, packaged, and delivered to military decision makers. Next, a feedback mechanism should exist whereby the decision maker can formulate questions to address to the producers of the information. The decision makers could ask for more information (deeper dive)

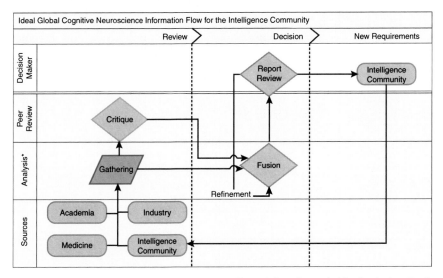

*Technology warning methodology detailed in the 2005 National Research Council report *Avoiding Surprise in an Era of Global Technology Advances*.

FIGURE 5-1 TIGER technology-warning method as one part of an overarching analytical information flow.

or clarification of specific issues presented in reporting. Finally, decision makers must identify topical areas requiring collection and analysis of information by the intelligence community.

As with weather forecasting, technology forecasting is measured in terms of probabilities, not certainties. Figure 5-2 is a notional diagram that illustrates some of the possibilities of technology-warning maturation. The abscissa of the diagram is time. It may be obvious, but it must be stated, that as analysts try to forecast farther into the future prediction becomes less accurate. By analogy, the afternoon weather forecast is more accurate than a 7-day forecast, which is more accurate than a 1-year forecast. The same difficulties will be apparent with neuroscience forecasting as analysts try to predict developments over the next 20 years. Figure 5-2 attempts to illustrate some considerations required in watching the development of cognitive neuroscience and related technologies.

In Figure 5-2, technology-warning levels are plotted on the ordinate of the diagram. The advancement of knowledge and technologies may have several trajectories, including linear and exponential, incremental, and nonlinear or crossover. Intelligence officers are often concerned with developing "trip wires" to avoid technology surprise. Trip wires are described as "observables" and "indicators" in *Avoiding Surprise* (NRC, 2005). To monitor these indicators of

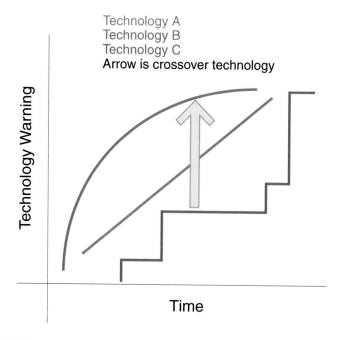

FIGURE 5-2 Technology warning over time. The graph depicts ways in which technology may be developed. Understanding the trajectory (incremental, exponential, and so on) in which specific types of technologies may develop could assist analysts in developing triggers and watching for crossovers.

technology warning (forecast changes or maximal potential) more correctly, some thought must be brought to bear on the journey that information may undergo on the way to increasing technology-warning levels; that is, the path must be studied, as well as the end point. Some things may be on a linear trajectory (Technology A in Figure 5-2) or an exponential trajectory (Technology B in Figure 5-2) similar to Moore's law of transistors doubling or increasing in magnetic resonance imaging (MRI) magnet size (Lloyd, 2000). Other types of science and technology warning concerns will develop in quantum or step functions (Technology C in Figure 5-2). Still other technologies will be crossover technologies (indicated by the yellow arrow in Figure 5-2). These were called innovation or integration events in *Avoiding Surprise* (NRC, 2005). Crossover technologies, such as the use of a cellular telephone in an improvised explosive device (IED), are difficult to predict and often represent extreme force multipliers.[1]

---

[1]A force multiplier is a capability that, when added to and used by a combat force, substantially increases the combat potential of that force and thus enhances the probability of mission accomplishment.

Most advances in cognitive neuroscience and related technologies will have dual uses. Pressures leading to advances will come from the pull of medical necessity and the push of science and technology advancement. Large state-funded programs are possible, but so is the use of new (or existing) technology in an innovation or integration. As cognitive neuroscience and related technologies become more pervasive, using technology for nefarious purposes becomes easier. Moreover, the triggers and observables become less obvious to the analyst and the collector. For example, a program using specialized equipment, such as that outlined on the Australia Group List of Biological Agents for Export Control, may or may not be applicable.[2] However, the types of experiments being done may be more telling than the type of equipment needed. The same equipment might be needed for medical and for disruptive neuropsychopharmacological experiments. It could be asked, What types of experiments are being done? How are the experiments being controlled and monitored, and why were they chosen? How would human experimentation be conducted outside accepted informed-consent limits?

MARKET DRIVERS OF COGNITIVE NEUROSCIENCE AND RELATED TECHNOLOGIES AS INDICATORS OF THE DEMAND FOR COTS TECHNOLOGIES

Overview

The military and intelligence community can forecast some aspects of how applied cognitive neuroscience technology might threaten the national security of the United States by tracking market drivers. Market drivers in this context are specific groups of neurotechnology consumers that create demand for development and delivery of applied cognitive neuroscience technology goods and services.[3] The applied cognitive neuroscience technology consumer landscape, for the purposes of this report, is categorized into three segments:

• *Health.* Customers are seeking help in addressing mental illness, brain disease, and injury;
• *Enhancement.* Customers do not possess a diagnosable neurological disorder but are seeking some cognitive performance advantage or want to prevent a probable decline; and

---

[2]For additional information, see Australia Group Web site, http://www.australiagroup.net/en/biological_agents.html. Last accessed on March 25, 2008.

[3]The report entitled *The Neurotechnology Industry 2007 Report: Drugs, Devices and Diagnostics for the Brain and Nervous System: Market Analysis and Strategic Investment Guide of the Global Neurological Disease and Psychiatric Illness Markets* from NeuroInsights provides a comprehensive breakdown of the current market drivers. For additional information, see Neuroinsights' Web site at http://www.neuroinsights.com/marketreports.html. Last accessed on January 24, 2008. The approach taken in this report segments the marketplace differently to comply with the statement of task.

• *Degradation.* Customers seek advantage by degrading, temporarily or permanently, the cognitive abilities of others.

There are dramatic differences in the motivations and sizes of these customer segments. The health market represents all the customers that would benefit from diagnosis, treatment, and cures for a mental illness or brain disorder. This market has been documented to be dramatically underserved in the United States and the world. Only about one-third of the potential market is actually served, leading to the two related conclusions: (1) the market has not reached its full potential and (2) the direct and indirect cost burden to the customers (and their governments) might change dramatically.[4]

Estimates vary on the potential revenue of the neurotechnology health market, but a reasonable estimate can be bounded by current revenue reports (as the low estimate) and total impact or cost burden (as the high estimate). Cost burden estimates include the cost of products and services as well as the indirect cost of no treatment. Total neurotechnology company revenue is about $120 billion; whereas total economic burden in the United States is on the order of $1 trillion per year and the world burden is about twice that.[5]

NIMH has stated that over 50 percent of Americans will suffer from a mental disorder in their lifetime. But the ability of this consumer group to pay for or get access to diagnosis, treatment, and cures constrains the health market segment. In other words, the demand exceeds the market's ability to provide goods and services in this segment.

The enhancement segment is largely underground, but growing. For example, healthy consumers cannot legally get a prescription to improve their attention or memory. However, there is significant anecdotal information that healthy people do take Alzheimer medication (Aricept), medication to treat narcolepsy (modafinil), and medication to treat attention deficit disorder (Ritalin) to improve performance. Sleep and wake medications, e.g., zolpidem and armodafinil, respectively, as products for enhancement represent a pharmaceutical market of over $5 billion. This market is generally more acceptable because one can be otherwise healthy and get a prescription. In many cases, the enhancement market is served by the off-label use of products and services created for the health market.

There are not good estimates for the potential revenue of the enhancement segment. Dramatic policy, ethical, and cultural changes will have to occur before this market becomes transparent and can grow quickly in the United States. But it is clear that the aging U.S. population will be a significant driver for this market.

---

[4]For detailed statistics, see the National Institute of Mental Health Web site at http://www.nimh. nih.gov/health/topics/statistics/index.shtml. Last accessed on January 18, 2008.

[5]For additional information, see the World Health Organization Web site at http://www.who.int/ healthinfo/bod/en/index.html for additional information. Last accessed on January 18, 2008.

The neurotechnology degradation market segment is completely underground with only speculative information available.[6] This cognitive weapons market does exist (e.g. the fentanyl derivative used in the 2002 Moscow theatre hostage crisis (Wax et al., 2003), and there is demand in the market from government agencies. There is potential for products that are developed for the health and enhancement markets to be misused in the degradation market—for example, using TMS to cause seizures (Pascual-Leone et al., 2002; NRC, 2003).

Finding 5-1. International market forces and global public demand have created an impetus for neuropsychopharmacology and neurotechnology research that will lead to new technologies and drugs, particularly in areas of cognition and performance, that will include off-label uses. Off-label drug use can alert intelligence analysts to compounds, methods of administration, or risk factors that may be unknown in civilian or military medicine and can help identify profiles of unanticipated effects.

The Search for New and Patentable Neurophysiological Agents

There are important U.S. and international market incentives for research activities in neuropsychopharmacology. No currently marketed drugs, psychotherapeutic or otherwise, are curative for mental illnesses; all have limited therapeutic efficacy, and all have undesired side effects. But the fact that many currently marketed drugs are or have been major sources of profit for the ethical pharmaceutical industry creates a market emphasis on finding new patentable entities. Additionally, analysts in a number of disciplines have predicted large increases in the prevalence of some disorders (e.g., Alzheimer's disease) that currently have few treatment options. This creates another strong market impetus.

One perhaps underappreciated feature of neuropsychopharmacology mentioned above further strengthens the market impetus. Few, if any, current psychotherapeutic drugs were designed or developed on the basis of an understanding of the psychopathology or the pathoetiology of the target disorder. Achievement of molecular- or organism-level understanding of pathophysiology of brain diseases will create enormous opportunities for drug discovery and development. Furthermore, the likelihood that some of these new drugs will exploit heretofore unknown mechanisms or brain functions creates opportunities for patentable pharmaceuticals. Any real advance in understanding of human behavior or brain disease could lead rapidly to truly new types of drugs, which could present potential positive or negative threats.

---

[6]For listings of neurotoxic agents and effects, see the Federation of American Scientists' Web site at http://www.fas.org/biosecurity/resource/lists.htm. Last accessed on January 24, 2008.

Market Barriers and How the Drivers May Change

Consumer demand drives the market, but markets always have constraints, both internal (consumer driven) and external (ethics, culture and government). The expansion and reduction of a market can be altered by changes such as new products, changes in regulations, or consumer awareness to name a few. The neurotechnology markets are highly influenced by the ethical, regulatory, political, and cultural environment.

This section looks at potential changes in the three categories listed above (health, enhancement and degradation) and then introduces two additional markets that could appear in strength in the future, the illegal and forced treatment neurotechnology markets.

Health Market

As stated earlier, there is a great deal of pent-up demand in the health market because of access and cost barriers. And overall demand for pharmaceuticals to treat mental illness and many physical diseases is moderated by the associated ineffectiveness or the side effects associated with many of the treatments. In the NIH CATIE schizophrenia study, approximately 70 percent of the patients did not do well on their first drug and had to be switched to a new drug. Customers seeking better health are often unsatisfied by the existing products—there is demand for improved and more cost-effective prevention and treatments.

One barrier to the expansion of the health market is the stigma associated with mental illness.[7] Social attitudes, ethics, and government policy remain major limiting factors. It has been a difficult battle to approve the Mental Health Parity Act of 2007 so that mental illness is viewed as a disease of the brain instead of a lifestyle choice or poor parenting. As awareness improves and health insurance broadens its payments for mental illness/brain disease, there could be as much as a doubling in treatment and associated revenue.

A significant barrier to market growth is the substantial investment of money and time needed to develop a drug for brain disease that is effective. On average, it takes almost 10 years and $500 million to take a neuropharmaceutical to market; however, new drug development could be aided by new technologies and processes, the market could advance more rapidly. Changes in related fields, such as genetics and neuroinformatics may be able to impact this process.

There is promise that once neuroimaging is used effectively in the development and evaluation of drug treatments, there could be radical changes in the health market. First, diagnostic imaging tools may be able to provide an objective, quantifiable diagnosis of a disease or illness and then second, they may allow for some level of prevention if diagnosis can occur earlier and then third, the treat-

---

[7]For additional information, see the Surgeon General's Web site at http://www.surgeongeneral. gov/library/mentalhealth/chapter1/sec1.html#roots_stigma. Last accessed on January 18, 2008.

ment could be more specific to the individual. Early and accurate diagnosis could lead to treatments with fewer side effects.

A factor that can potentially grow the neurotechnology health market is the advent of neuroinformatics. Diagnosis, prevention, treatment and then cure of brain injury and disease will benefit from better use of the complex array of information associated with a given health problem. Patient information, behavior, genetics, and image data can be combined to better understand the individual aspects of the affliction. As mentioned before, neuroinformatics may well enable a shortened development cycle for new drugs and treatment regimens.

Finding 5-2. Neurotechnology products may be dual use. Products intended for the health market can be used in the enhancement and degradation markets. Additionally, the product life cycle can be shunted because of the nature of the enhancement and degradation markets.

Enhancement Market

The neurotechnology enhancement market is analogous to the athletic performance enhancement market. People will make the choice to take illegal and off-label prescription neuropharmaceuticals even if they do not know the side effects or believe that the side effects are worth the potential enhancement. This controversial market will grow dramatically if evidence becomes available that a specific drug is consistently effective in improving performance. However, if this market expansion does occur, it is likely that current attitudes will prevail and result in use being squelched through policy and law. History shows that prohibition will not work to stop consumption of a banned product and that the government that takes the path of prohibition will invest in methods to diagnose the abuse.

In addition to off-label use of FDA approved drugs and devices, there are enhancement products available that are not subject to FDA approval. These include software products and vitamin supplements. In almost all cases, the effectiveness of these products has not been established with a clinical trial-like process, but their popularity is increasing (Vollset and Ueland, 2005). The software products are focused on enhancing neural plasticity and delaying the effects of aging. In some cases, they include direct neural feedback using EEG. This nascent market could grow rapidly because of the ease of developing new products and the lack of clear regulations. An interesting off-label use of an inexpensive iontophoresis dose controller is as a transcranial direct current stimulation system, or tDCS.[8] tDCS enhances certain cognitive functions (Antal et al., 2006).

---

[8]For additional information, see the IOMED Web site at http://www.iomed.com. Last accessed on January 18, 2008.

TABLE 5-1 Current Drugs Used in New Ways or For New Targets and New Types of Drug Entities

Target of Agent for Change	Current Agents That Might Achieve Aim or Part of Aim
Memory, learning, cognitive speed	Various drugs, stem cell reparative therapy, nanoneural networks
Alertness and impulse control	Stimulants, modafinil, ampakines, antidepressants
Mood, anxiety, and self perception	Beta blockers, selective serotonin re-uptake inhibitors
Creativity	Transcranial magnetic stimulation
Trust, empathy, and moral decision making	Oxytocin, testosterone suppression
Sleep and wake medications	Zolpidem, armodafinil

SOURCE: Hughes (2007). ©2007 by Elsevier. Reprinted with permission.

The 65 and over population is expected to double in the next 25 years. This shift to an older population, with 20 percent of the population over the age of 65 by 2020, will increase demand for enhancement neurotechnology. Much of the market growth could be limited to non-FDA controlled products because of the associated policy issues. Public and medical demand for enhancement or a competitive edge may create market impetus in many areas. This public climate is illustrated by sources as respectable as a 2006 report in the Harvard Crimson about student demand for stimulants,[9] a 2008 NYTimes.com report about professional baseball players claiming medical exemptions for stimulant use,[10] and a 2003 Fortune magazine report suggesting memory pills for a competitive edge.[11] Development areas that may respond to such market incentives include cognition and mentation in all their forms (arousal, attention, cognition, learning, memory, motivation, among others), movement and performance (strength, speed, stamina, motor learning, among others), and mood (anxiety, depression, craving, emotional memories, among others).

As noted earlier, development of new agents for such uses could result in drug entities that change cognition, performance, or mood in unexpected, currently unavailable ways. The examples in Table 5-1 drawn from Hughes (2007) suggest both current drugs used in new ways or for new targets and new types of drug entities.

---

[9]For additional information, see http://www.thecrimson.com/article.aspx?ref=513261. Last accessed on January 23, 2008.

[10]For additional information, see http://www.nytimes.com/2008/01/19/sports/baseball/19stimulants.html?_r=1&ref=sports&oref=slogin. Last accessed on January 23, 2008.

[11]For additional information, see http://money.cnn.com/magazines/fortune/fortune_archive/2003/05/12/342287/index.htm. Last accessed on January 23, 2008.

Actual progress, or at least actual changes, in such development programs may accelerate as drug developers attempt to define drugs with more targeted psychological or cognitive effects. As discussed in another context, much research on "cognition enhancers" has sought broadly acting drugs. Programs that target narrower, more specific, effects on cognition may be more interesting and warrant attention. For example, drugs that appear (at least initially) to have effects concentrated in one area, such as speed of learning, accuracy of retention, selective retention or selective forgetting (as of traumatic memories), expanded attention span, and social cognition, might deserve particular attention. Such agents might warrant attention for both their risks and their ability to enhance performance and safety of the individual warfighter.

Drug entities developed to have increased selectivity of effects on cognition or performance might conceivably be integrated into enemy military programs. Their adoption by a military force, for example, might be facilitated both by their targeted effects and by possible reductions in side-effect profiles. Agents now used to enhance cognition or performance can pose safety risks to warfighters that include abuse, misuse (e.g., excessive doses or too frequent use), unintended consequences, unexpected interactions with situations, and alterations in social behavior. Indeed, drug entities with reduced side-effect profiles could achieve greater use, independent of increased selectivity of action.

Adoption of such agents by medical practitioners, patients, and/or portions of the general public will be influenced by important social and cultural forces, as discussed elsewhere in this report. One force that might warrant particular analysis is inflated or frankly bogus marketing claims for specificity, effectiveness, or safety made by sources in private, government and/or academic sectors.

Degradation Market

The development of a more humane way of fighting a war by using cognitive weapons could dramatically change the degradation neurotechnology market. Pills instead of bullets. The fear that this approach to fighting war might be developed will be justification for developing countermeasures to possible cognitive weapons. This escalation might lead to innovations that could cause this market area to expand rapidly. Tests would need to be developed to determine if a soldier had been harmed by a cognitive weapon. And there would be a need for a prophylactic of some sort. If a particularly effective degradation product is developed that has few side effects, escalation of this market will be self-fulfilling. The concept of torture could also be altered by products in this market. It is possible that someday there could be a technique developed to extract information from a prisoner that does not have any lasting side effects. Recently, it has been documented in a small study that tDCS delays a person's ability to tell a lie (Priori et al., 2007).

Finding 5-3. Neurotechnology products developed specifically for the enhancement and degradation markets may not be subject to the same development and distribution/access constraints that apply to the health market. Safety, social, ethical, and legal constraints may not apply in countries where regulation is less rigorous.

Forced Treatment Market

There are instances where it might be possible in the future to control a person's behavior through the application of drugs or electromagnetic devices. It is estimated that about 25 percent of prisoners are mentally ill. There are currently significant efforts to identify the brain/biological basis of certain types of criminal behavior. What if certain types of criminal behavior had a biological/brain basis and could be prevented with treatment? Some cultures or governments may determine that forced treatment gives them a competitive advantage by reducing the cost burden of disease and illness. This has occurred in the United States for things like tuberculosis. The limiting factor for this market to grow is resolution of the related ethical issues. For example, the Mind Research Network has collected the neuroimaging and genetic data on over 300 prisoners using a mobile MRI facility and has a goal of collecting a thousand subjects by 2009. As stated in Chapter 4, current guidelines for ethical recruitment and participation of human volunteers in research generally prohibit participation by prisoners, due to actual or potential coercion risk (IOM, 2006).

TECHNOLOGY ASSESSMENTS: NEUROPSYCHOPHARMACOLOGY

Current scientific understanding of neuropsychopharmacology suggests types of drugs whose appearance in national or international research or commercial arenas might pose predictable threats to U.S. warfighters. One type of identifiable threat might be development of antagonists for drug entities that currently have no antagonists, such as an antagonist for ethanol. Such an antagonist could allow adversaries to protect their own warfighters against an agent that is widely dispersed (for example, in gas, in aerosols, in drinking water, or by high-altitude delivery). Another type would be the coupling of known agents with unexpected routes of administration, doses, or personnel protective agents. A known example is the aerosol use of fentanyl during the Russian hostage-taking (an instance of all three surprises).

Other threats could arise from training of warfighters to operate under new pharmacological conditions. An adversary could train warfighters to operate under the influence of chemical agents that ordinarily disrupt performance or could modify warfighters to resist such agents. Such resistance could be conferred by means of changes in genetics, physiology, training, pharmacology, or psychology. Either tactic could allow adversaries to operate while chemical agents are dispersed against civilians or U.S. combatants. Warfighters might also be trained or modified (as above) to detect their own degraded performance more accurately and take corrective action (such as taking a drug or calling for backup). Drugs that are not usually thought of as having psychological or performance effects might be used by warfighters or civilians as countermeasures against emerging technologies for detection of deception or cognition. A perhaps far-fetched example would be use of such a drug as Botox® to defeat systems for detection of facial expressions.

Particularly important changes in drug development may arise from the emerging field of personalized medicine. It has been suggested that developments in understanding of genetic control of physiology and psychology will improve "individualization" of drugs and their effects. Drugs tailored to a person's genetic, psychological, or situational conditions might, for example, increase cognition or performance and reduce disruptive or mission-incompatible side effects. Such developments may also create drug entities that have the capacity to alter human functioning genetically. For example, basic research on the genetics of brain function may create the possibility of genetic memory enhancement—use of genetic technology to change expression of molecules involved in memory or other cognitive functions. Research in mice has provided "proof of principle" that overexpression of brain proteins may enhance memory: these research programs have targeted the *N*-methyl-D-aspartate 2B receptor (Tang et al., 1999; Bliss, 1999), the brain-growth GAP-43 protein (Routtenberg et al., 2000), and type 1 adenylyl cyclase (Wang et al., 2004). Development of pharmacological agents to mimic effects of "memory genes" might warrant considerable attention. In all of those areas, technology surprise may well stem from an adversary's willingness to use means that U.S. warfighters would not use because of ethical values and policy constraints.

As discussed in Chapter 2, the blood-brain barrier (BBB) can be thought of as an anatomical defensive perimeter that keeps substances from entering the brain. New technologies, particularly nanotechnologies, will enable unparalleled access to the brain. Nanotechnologies can also exploit existing transport mechanisms to transmit substances into the brain in analogy with the Trojan horse. Advances in nanotechnology and BBB pharmacology—for example, advances in chemotherapeutics; antimicrobials; treatment of Alzheimer disease; and reversals of cerebrovascular insults—will allow chemical disruption of the BBB. Additionally, increased experimentation with neuropeptides will have profound implications for the neuropsychopharmacological modulation of behavior. See Charts 5-1 to 5-4 for examples of the committee's application of the technology warning methodology to the area of neuropsychopharmacology.

CHART 5-1 Use of Neuropsychological Agents as Incapacitants

Technology	Triggers and Observables
Aerosols of opioids serve as excellent incapacitants; reversal agents and premedications can be administered to protect soldiers. Russia deployed this technology in the Moscow Dubrovka Theater in 2002. The agents were probably fentanyl derivatives and may have included inhalation anesthetics (Wax et al., 2003).	Future military deployments and/or training by other countries should be observed. In addition, medicinal chemical developments of other countries should be observed for military applications of medical pharmacology, with particular attention to more potent fentanyl derivatives and inhalation anesthetics. Attention should also be given to technologies that would allow aerosol release in building ventilation systems.

Accessibility	Maturity	Consequence
Level 3	Warning	This technology is asymmetrical in that the U.S. military is not believed to have it, whereas Russia is known to have it and to have deployed it. The consequence of releasing material would be nonlethal incapacitation of U.S. operators or assets. A small number of enemy operators could rapidly incapacitate a larger number of U.S. forces without engaging in combat. Once incapacitated, the blue forces could be killed or captured by the red forces that had been pretreated with antidote.

CHART 5-2 Nanotechnologies or Gas-Phase Technologies That Allow Dispersal of Highly Potent Chemicals over Wide Areas

Technology	Triggers and Observables
Pharmacological agents are not used as weapons of mass effect, because their large-scale deployment is impractical; it is currently impossible to get an effective dose to a combatant. However, technologies that could be available in the next 20 years would allow dispersal of agents in delivery vehicles that would be analogous to a pharmacological cluster bomb or a land mine.	Triggers to watch for would be development of such technologies for agricultural or pesticide purposes. Precedents exist for using toxins as weapons delivered by ingestion, transdermally, or by inhalation. Analysts should watch for development of standardized delivery systems that can distribute small-molecule "payloads" over large areas, such as crop fields. Those delivery systems would protect agents from meteorological conditions and then release agents on contact with a soldier. Of particular concern would be a single delivery system that could be easily loaded with different agents, as warheads are switched in an artillery round. This type of system would allow easy crossover to nefarious purposes.

Accessibility	Maturity	Consequence
Level 2	Futures	The consequence of such a system would be an off-the-shelf small-molecule delivery system that could be leveraged against U.S. forces. Highly potent compounds could cause troop incapacitation or performance degradation. Coupling off-the-shelf agents with an off-the-shelf delivery system would create new threat opportunities against U.S. forces. Spreading agents that would be released on contact would deny U.S. military operations some strategic infrastructure or geographic positions.

CHART 5-3 Technologies for Highly Potent Blood-Pressure Agents or Sensory-Specific Pharmacological Targeting

Technology	Triggers and Observables
Existing pharmacological agents could be used in a nefarious way. An example would be currently used agents, such as alpha blockers, that would work quickly to drop blood pressure if delivered in high doses. In addition, anticholinergic agents could cause molecular changes that lead to temporary blindness.	The literature should be monitored for development of sympathomimetic and parasympatholytic drugs. Development may be revealed in basic chemical discovery and synthesis pathways. Antihypertensives continue to be of great pharmacological research and development interest. Clinical trials should be monitored closely, and reports of unknown or unrecognized incapacitants should be carefully analyzed.

Accessibility	Maturity	Consequence
Level 2	Futures	The consequence of development of these technologies would be an asymmetrical threat to U.S. troops. The consequence of releasing material would be nonlethal incapacitation of U.S. operators or assets. A small number of enemy operators could rapidly incapacitate a larger number of U.S. forces without engaging in combat. Once incapacitated, the U.S. forces could be killed or captured by enemy forces that had been pretreated with an antidote.

CHART 5-4 Drug-Delivery Systems Applied to the Blood-Brain Barrier

Technology	Triggers and Observables
New nanotechnologies have allowed molecular conjugation or encapsulation that may permit unprecedented access to the brain.	Triggers and observables include open-source publications and collaboration between pharmaceutical companies and industrial fabricators of nanotechnologies. Research and development will continue because of the need for new neuropharmaceuticals. This is a subject of broad international interest and should be monitored to maintain U.S. awareness of these technologies as related to the blood-brain barrier. Human trials with regard to drug delivery to the central nervous system should also be monitored closely because it will be required for technology maturation.

Accessibility	Maturity	Consequence
Level 2	Warning	Increased access to the brain by drugs that cross the blood-brain barrier would allow increased potency of therapeutics. Brain injury remains a scourge of the warfighter; better treatment by military medical personnel would be of extreme benefit to our troops. Not only would successful treatment for injuries increase morale, but it would allow for return of highly trained personnel to active duty. On the disruptive side, if an adversary were able to breach the blood-brain barrier, warfighters could be rapidly incapacitated. That could be done by covertly assaulting troops, and the result could range from severe incapacitation to death.

TECHNOLOGY ASSESSMENTS: DISTRIBUTED HUMAN-MACHINE SYSTEMS AND COMPUTATIONAL BIOLOGY

One example of a potential threat in the category of distributed human-machine systems and computational biology is a computational cognitive framework. Computers are used widely and successfully to store, recall, and process information, but they do those things very differently from humans. Although modeling the whole brain in the next 2 decades is highly unlikely, it is not unreasonable to imagine that substantial subsystems could be modeled. Moreover, increasingly sophisticated cognitive systems will probably be constructed in that period that, although not aiming to mimic processes in the brain, could perform similar tasks adequately enough to be useful, especially in constrained situations. Making up in part for the lack of years of "experience" that constitutes an important basis of much of human intelligence, intelligent systems are increasingly using the Internet to assist in their training. In the next 2 decades, one can easily imagine artificial cognitive systems that will be increasingly capable of complex reasoning that, in combination with human capabilities, can exploit an incredibly large amount of knowledge and substantially advance the ability of human analysts to monitor large amounts of information and to formulate and test credible hypotheses.

A second example of a potential threat in the category of distributed human-machine systems and computational biology stems from physiomimetic computing hardware. With the exception of a few small-scale endeavors, the computational-cognition community has essentially been confined to using large-scale general-purpose computers for almost all its modeling and simulation efforts. However, the digital computers have evolved through a history of solving computational problems that lend themselves well to the notion of precise logic or well-structured probabilistic or statistical models. The brain is inherently different, with its neurons and other components acting more as analog devices with a continuous set of values and a complex set of connections. It is possible that one could make important advances in artificial cognitive modeling by constructing a computer based on analog circuits that would address many of today's modeling and simulation challenges. Such a computer could perhaps be much smaller than today's digital computers and be easy for the United States or its adversaries to construct (Watson, 1997; Konar; 2000; Von Neumann, 2000; Giles, 2001; Arbib, 2003; Siegelmann, 2003; Schemmel et al., 2004; Trautteur and Tamburrini, 2007; Mills, 2008).

A third example stems from microscopic magnetic detectors. Precision detection of magnetic fields in atomic devices is quickly becoming a mainstream technology. Previously, superconducting quantum interference devices (SQUIDs) were the primary means of precision magnetic-field detection, but the necessity of having ultralow temperature has prevented SQUIDs from becoming an inexpensive, simple-to-use technology. New microscience and nanoscience technologies that will enable small precision magnetometers (measured in millimeters) are emerging. They could enable dramatic increases in the number of sensors (and, similarly, spatial resolution) and the portability of measurement devices. Such changes could revolutionize neuroimaging.

A fourth example is a brain-machine interface (BMI) for the control of weapons systems. With breakthroughs in training and the detection of brain activity for BMIs to the required level of complexity and specificity, virtually any conceivable weapons system could be controlled by this means. Basic research would need to be performed to determine the ultimate range of physiological potential and the limitations of such interfaces. Even if this range of performance were found to be feasible, it would remain to be demonstrated that BMIs are superior to conventional methods for controlling computing functions and robotic vehicles. With respect to the use of brain scanning in combat risk-assessment devices, it has been suggested that a weapons system could indicate potentially hostile forces as candidate targets while passing over noncombatants. Functional neuroimaging technology can already reliably discriminate between men and women, and it seems possible that this kind of capability could be extended to take other simple discriminators into account. However, it would require exceptional advances in technology to have the capability to discriminate reliably between combatants with potentially hostile intent and noncombatants without hostile intent, and such a capability may ultimately be infeasible given the wide range of individual differences and the high consequences of misidentification.

A final example would be the development of sophisticated distributed human-machine systems that are capable of greatly enhancing the cognitive and physical performance of human warfighters or allowing them to coordinate the actions of autonomous systems effectively. See Charts 5-5 to 5-8 for examples of the committee's application of the technology warning methodology to the areas of computational biology and distributed human-machine systems.

FINDINGS AND RECOMMENDATION

Finding 5-4. Rapid advances in cognitive neuroscience, as in science and technology in general, represent a major challenge to the IC. The IC does not have the internal capability to warn against scientific developments that could lead to major—even catastrophic—intelligence failures in the years ahead. An effective warning model must depend on continuous input from strong internal science and technology programs, strong interactive networks with outside scientific experts, and government decision makers who engage in the process and take it seriously as a driver of resources. All that remains a work in progress for the IC.

Technology warning in the IC today is hampered by several factors including the low priority it has among senior leaders; the paucity of resources invested by the community in internal science and technology capability; the continuing inadequate management attention to the needs of IC analysts; and the need to establish

CHART 5-5 Computational Cognitive Framework

Technology	Triggers and Observables
A computational cognitive framework that, in combination with human capabilities, can monitor and perform complex reasoning on large amounts of knowledge from the Internet.	• Research papers. • Commercial products. • Increased or unusual Web crawling.

Accessibility	Maturity	Consequence
Level 1	Watch	This technology would lead to important advances in the ability of human analysts to monitor large amounts of information and to formulate and test credible hypotheses.

CHART 5-6 Physiomimetic Computing Hardware

Technology	Triggers and Observables
Analogue "brain-like" computer that would enable a different approach to computational cognition.	• Substantial investment in analogue-computing hardware. • Revolutionary new algorithms that take advantage of the new hardware.

Accessibility	Maturity	Consequence
Level 3	Futures	Access to an artificial cognitive system at a very low price. This is a low-probability event, but such a system could provide both inexpensive intelligence and potentially an offensive-cyberwarfare capability.

CHART 5-7 Microscopic Magnetic Detectors

Technology	Triggers and Observables	
Millimeter-sized magnetic detectors that require volume under 0.5 cm³ and ultralow power.	New commercial products or research devices that would enable functional imaging in traditional application environments.	

Accessibility	Maturity	Consequence
Level 2	Alert	Imaging device with extreme portability and many more channels of data. It would give the developer a revolutionary advantage in understanding of neural behavior in realistic situations.

CHART 5-8 Sophisticated Distributed Human-Machine Systems

Technology	Triggers and Observables	
Software or robotic assistants for advanced sensor grids, control and coordination of unmanned autonomous systems, advanced command posts and intelligence analyst workbenches, coordination of joint or coalition operations, logistics, and information assurance.	• Research papers. • Commercial products.	

Accessibility	Maturity	Consequence
Level 2	Alert	This technology would greatly enhance the cognitive or physical performance of warfighters and decision-makers or allow them to coordinate the actions of autonomous systems with much-improved effectiveness.

close ongoing collaborations with analysts in other agencies, in the scientific community at large, the corporate world, and academia, where the IC can find the most advanced understanding of scientific trends and their implications.

Finding 5-5. The recommendations in this report to improve technology warning for cognitive neuroscience and related technologies are unlikely to succeed unless the following issues are addressed:

- Emphasizing science and technology as a priority for intelligence collection and analysis.
- Appointing and retaining accomplished IC professionals with advanced scientific and technical training to aid in the development of S&T collection strategies.
- Increasing external collaboration by the IC with the academic community. It should be noted that some components of the IC have made great strides in reaching out to the academic community.

Recommendation 5-1. The intelligence community should use a more centralized indication and warning process that involves analysis, requirement generation, and reporting. Engagement with the academic community is required and is good, but it is not now systematically targeted against foreign research.

REFERENCES

Arbib, Michael. 2003. *The Handbook of Brain Theory and Neural Networks*: Second Edition. MIT Press, Cambridge, MA.

Antal, A., M.A. Nitsche, and W. Paulus. 2006. Transcranial direct current stimulation and the visual cortex. *Brain Resolution Bulletin* 68(6):459-463.

Bliss, T.V.P. 1999. Neurobiology: Young receptors make smart mice. *Nature* 401(6748):25-27.

Giles, Jim. 2001. Think like a bee. *Nature* 410(6828):510-512.

Hughes, James. 2007. The struggle for a smarter world. *Futures* 39(8):942-954.

IOM (Institute of Medicine). 2006. *Ethical Considerations for Research Involving Prisoners.* Washington, D.C.: The National Academies Press. Available from http://www.iom.edu/CMS/3740/24594/35792.aspx.

Konar, Amit. 2000. *Artificial Intelligence and Soft Computing: Behavioral and Cognitive Modeling of the Human Brain.* Boca Raton, FL: CRC Press.

Lloyd, Seth. 2000. Ultimate physical limits to computation. *Nature* 406 (6788):1047-1054.

Mills, Jonathan. 2008. The nature of the extended analog computer. *Physica D: Nonlinear Phenomena* 237(9):1235-1256.

NRC (National Research Council). 2003. *The Polygraph and Lie Detection.* Washington, DC: The National Academies Press. Available from http://www.nap.edu/catalog.php?record_id=10420.

NRC. 2005. *Avoiding Surprise in an Era of Global Technology Advances.* Washington, DC: The National Academies Press.

Pascual-Leone, A., N.J. Davey, J. Rothwell, E.M. Wasseran, and B.K. Puri. 2002. *Handbook of Transcranial Magnetic Stimulation.* London: Arnold.

Priori, A., F. Mameli, F. Cogiamanian, S. Marceglia, M. Tiriticco, S. Mrakic-Sposta, R. Ferrucci, S. Zago, D. Polezzi, and G. Sartori. 2007. Lie specific involvement of dorsolateral prefrontal cortex in deception. *Cerebral Cortex* 18(2):451-455.

Routtenberg, Aryeh, Isabel Cantallops, Sal Zaffuto, Peter Serrano, and Uk Namgung. 2000. Enhanced learning after genetic overexpression of a brain growth protein. *Proceedings of the National Academy of Sciences U.S.A.* 97(13):7657-7662.

Schemmel, J., S. Hohmann, K. Meier, and F. Schurmann. 2004. A mixed-mode analog neural network using current-steering synapses. *Analog Integrated Circuits and Signal Processing* 38(2):233-244.

Siegelmann, H. 2003. Neural and super-Turing computing. *Minds and Machines* 13(1):103-114.

Tang, Ya-Ping, Eiji Shimizu, Gilles R. Dube, Claire Rampon, Geoffrey A. Kerchner, Min Zhuo, Guosong Liu, and Joe Z. Tsien. 1999. Genetic enhancement of learning and memory in mice. *Nature* 401(6748):25-27.

Trautteur, G., and G. Tamburrini. 2007. A note on discreteness and virtuality in analog computing. *Theoretical Computer Science* 371(1-2):106-114.

Vollset, Stein Emil, and Per Magne Ueland. 2005. B vitamins and cognitive function: Do we need more and larger trials? *American Journal of Clinical Nutrition* 81(5):951-952.

Von Neumann, John (updated by Paul M. Churchland and Patricia S. Churchland). 2000. *The Computer and the Brain*. New Haven, CT: Yale University Press.

Wang, Hongbing, Gregory D. Ferguson, Victor V. Pineda, Paige E. Cundiff, and Daniel R. Storm. 2004. Overexpression of type-1 adenylyl cyclase in mouse forebrain enhances recognition memory and LTP. *Nature Neuroscience* 7(6):635-642.

Watson, Andrew. 1997. Neuromorphic engineering: Why can't a computer be more like a brain? *Science* 277(5334):1934-1936.

Wax, P.M., C.E. Becker, and S.C. Curry. (2003). Unexpected "gas" casualties in Moscow: A medical toxicology perspective. *Annals of Emergency Medicine* 41(5):700-705.

Appendixes

Appendix A

Biographical Sketches of Committee Members

Christopher C. Green, *Chair,* is the assistant dean for Asia Pacific of the Wayne State School of Medicine (SOM) in Beijing, China. He is also a clinical fellow in neuroimaging/MRI in the Department of Diagnostic Radiology and the Department of Psychiatry and Behavioral Neurosciences of the SOM and the Detroit Medical Center (DMC). His medical specialties are brain imaging, forensic medicine and toxicology, and neurophysiology, and his personal medical practice is in the differential diagnoses of neurodegenerative disease. He has served and continues to serve on many government advisory groups and private sector corporate boards of directors. Immediately prior to his current position, he was executive director for emergent technology research for the SOM/DMC. From 1985 through 2004 he was executive director, Global Technology Policy, and chief technology officer for General Motors' Asia-Pacific Operations. His career at General Motors included positions as head, Biomedical Sciences Research, and executive director, General Motors Research Laboratory for Materials and Environmental Sciences. His distinguished career with the CIA extended from 1969 to 1985 as a senior division analyst and assistant national intelligence officer for science and technology. His Ph.D. is from the University of Colorado Medical School in neurophysiology, and his M.D. is from the Autonomous City University in El Paso, Texas/Monterey, Mexico, with honors. He also holds the National Intelligence Medal and is a fellow in the American Academy of Forensic Sciences. Dr. Green is a current member of the National Research Council's Standing Committee on Technology Insight—Gauge, Evaluate, and Review (TIGER).

Diane E. Griffin, *Vice Chair,* is a member of the National Academy of Sciences and the Institute of Medicine and is professor and chair of the Department of

Molecular Microbiology and Immunology at Johns Hopkins Bloomberg School of Public Health. She earned a biology degree from Augustana College, followed by an M.D. (1968) and a Ph.D. from Stanford University. She interned at Stanford University Hospital between 1968 and 1970, before beginning her career at Johns Hopkins as a postdoctoral fellow in virology and infectious disease in 1970. After completing her postdoctoral work, she was named an assistant professor of medicine and neurology. Since then, she has held the positions of associate professor, professor, and now professor and chair. She served as an investigator in the Howard Hughes Medical Institute from 1973 to 1979. Dr. Griffin's research interest includes alphaviruses and acute encephalitis. She is also working on virus infection and its effects on immune responses. Dr. Griffin is the principal investigator on a variety of grants from the National Institutes of Health and the Bill and Melinda Gates Foundation. She is a past president of the American Society for Microbiology of the American Society for Virology and the Association of Medical School Microbiology Chairs. She is the author or coauthor of a number of scholarly papers and articles. Dr. Griffin is a current member of the TIGER standing committee.

James J. Blascovich is a professor of psychology at the University of California, Santa Barbara. Dr. Blascovich earned a B.S. in psychology at Loyola University of Chicago and a Ph.D. in social psychology at the University of Nevada, Reno. He held academic positions at the University of Nevada, Reno, Marquette University, and SUNY at Buffalo before coming to the University of California, Santa Barbara. Dr. Blascovich directs the Research Center for Virtual Environments and Behavior and is a past president of both the Society for Personality and Social Psychology and the Society of Experimental Social Psychology. He is a member of the Academy of Behavioral Medicine Research, a charter fellow of the Association of Psychological Science, and a fellow of the American Psychological Association. Dr. Blascovich was awarded the Inaugural Australasian Social Psychology Society/Society of Personality and Social Psychology Teaching Fellowship as well as an Erskine Fellowship and a Science Prestige Lectureship at the University of Canterbury in New Zealand. He won the Gordon Allport Prize Intergroup Relations Prize for 2007. He has also received the Chancellor's Award for Excellence in Undergraduate Research at the University of California, Santa Barbara. Dr. Blascovich has served on several grant review panels and was appointed to the National Research Council's Committee to Evaluate the Scientific Evidence on the Polygraph. He chaired the Committee on Opportunities in Basic Research in the Behavioral and Social Sciences for the military. He has served on many editorial boards of journals, including *Psychological Science* and the *Journal of Personality and Social Psychology*, *Psychological Inquiry*, *Media Psychology*, and *Presence*. In addition to receiving periodic funding from the National Institutes of Health, Dr. Blascovich's research has received continuous funding from the National Science Foundation for more than 18 years.

Jeffrey M. Bradshaw is a senior research scientist at the Florida Institute for Human and Machine Cognition where he leads the research group developing the KAoS policy and domain services framework. Formerly, he led research groups at The Boeing Company and the Fred Hutchinson Cancer Research Center. He has been a Fulbright senior scholar at the European Institute for Cognitive Sciences and Engineering in Toulouse, France; an honorary visiting researcher at the Center for Intelligent Systems and their Applications and AIAI at the University of Edinburgh, Scotland; a visiting professor at the Institut Cognitique at the University of Bordeaux; is former chair of ACM SIGART; and former chair of the RIACS Science Council for NASA Ames Research Center. Dr. Bradshaw sat on the external advisory board for the Next Generation Intelligent Systems Grand Challenge at Sandia National Laboratories and is a current member of the Technical Committee for IEEE Systems, Man and Cybernetics. Recently, he served as co-program chair for Intelligent User Interfaces and as program vice chair of the 2008 IEEE International Conference on Distributed Human-Machine Systems. Dr. Bradshaw serves on the board of directors of the International Foundation for Autonomous Agents and Multiagent Systems and is a member of the Parametric Human Consortium. He is on the editorial board of the *Journal of Autonomous Agents and Multi-Agent Systems*, the *Web Semantics Journal, Schedae Informaticae,* and the *Web Intelligence Journal,* and was formerly on the board of the *Knowledge Acquisition Journal* and the *International Journal of Human-Computer Studies.* He led the DARPA- and NASA-funded ITAC study team "Software Agents for the Warfighter" and participated in NASA Blue Sky Study Groups for the "Human-Centered Vision of Mars Exploration" and for the "Small Pressurized Rover."

Scott C. Bunce is an assistant professor of psychiatry at Drexel University College of Medicine, and holds a joint position in Drexel's School of Biomedical Engineering, Science & Health Systems. Dr. Bunce received doctorates in clinical and personality psychology from the University of Michigan and completed his postdoctoral training in the Department of Psychiatry at Michigan. He is the director of Drexel's Clinical Neuroscience Research Unit (CNSRU), a laboratory that investigates a broad range of topics related to affective and cognitive neuroscience using noninvasive measures of brain function. A particular focus of the CNSRU in recent years has been the development and implementation of functional near-infrared spectroscopy (fNIRS), an optical technology that allows inexpensive and portable cortical neuroimaging. In collaboration with Drexel's optical imaging team in the School of Biomedical Engineering, Dr. Bunce has received numerous grants to investigate the utility of fNIRS for monitoring and augmenting cognition, e.g., attention and memory, and for credibility assessment/ deception detection. A motivating interest of the optical imaging team is to transition fNIRS-based functional neuroimaging into clinical and research applications that are not practical for other neuroimaging modalities. In addition to his research, Dr. Bunce is an active clinician and educator, and has focused on the development of innovative strategies to provide mental health care and addiction treatment to HIV+ patients.

John Gannon is vice president for global analysis, a new line of business within BAE Systems Information Technology. Dr. Gannon joins BAE Systems after serving as staff director of the House Homeland Security Committee, the first new committee established by Congress in more than 30 years. In 2002-2003, he was a team leader in the White House's Transitional Planning Office for the Department of Homeland Security. He served previously in the most senior analytic positions in the intelligence community, including as CIA's director of European analysis, deputy director for intelligence, chairman of the National Intelligence Council, and assistant director of Central Intelligence for Analysis and Production. In the private sector, he developed the analytic workforce for Intellibridge Corporation, a Web-based provider of outsourced analysis for government and corporate clients. Dr. Gannon served as a naval officer in southeast Asia and later in several Naval Reserve commands, retiring as a captain. He holds a Ph.D. from Washington University in St. Louis. He is an adjunct professor in the National Security Studies Program at Georgetown University. Dr. Gannon is a current member of the TIGER standing committee.

Michael Gazzaniga, a member of the Institute of Medicine, is the first director of the Sage Center for the Study of the Mind at the University of California, Santa Barbara. He received his Ph.D. in psychobiology from the California Institute of Technology. In 1992, he became the director of the Center for Neuroscience at the University of California, Davis. Through his extensive work with split-brain patients, Dr. Gazzaniga has made important advances in our understanding of functional lateralization in the human brain and of how the cerebral hemispheres communicate with one another. His research is well known not only to clinical and basic science circles but also to the lay public. He captured the main features of this work in his widely acclaimed book *The Social Brain*. His book *Mind Matters* served as an introduction to problems in mental disorders. About his book *Nature's Mind* the *New York Times* said it would do for brain research what Stephen Hawking had done for cosmology. His 1995 book, *The Cognitive Neurosciences*, featured the work of 92 scientists. It is now recognized as the sourcebook for the field and is in its third edition. He has just published another book, *Human: The Science Behind What Makes Us Unique*. Dr. Gazzaniga is the president of the Cognitive Neuroscience Institute, which he founded in 1982, and is the editor in chief emeritus of the *Journal of Cognitive Neuroscience*, which he also founded. In 1997, Dr. Gazzaniga was elected to the American Academy of Arts and Sciences. He also has been elected president of the American Psychological Society and also serves on the President's Council on Bioethics.

Elizabeth Loftus, a member of the National Academy of Sciences, is distinguished professor at the University of California, Irvine. She holds faculty positions in three departments (Psychology and Social Behavior; Criminology, Law, and Society; and Cognitive Sciences) and is also a fellow of the Center for the Neurobiology of Learning and Memory, She was also recently appointed professor of law. She received a Ph.D. in psychology from Stanford University. Since then, she has published 22 books, including the award-winning *Eyewitness Testimony*, and over 475 scientific articles. Dr. Loftus's research over the last 30 years has focused on the malleability of human memory. She has been recognized for this research with five honorary doctorates and election to the Royal Society of Edinburgh and the American Philosophical Society. She is past president of the Association for Psychological Science, the Western Psychological Association, and the American Psychology-Law Society.

Gregory J. Moore is a neuroscientist, physician, engineer, and physicist with over 15 years of experience in the development and application of advanced neuroimaging tools to investigate the brain and brain illness. After obtaining a Ph.D. at the Massachusetts Institute of Technology, where he developed advanced nuclear magnetic resonance imaging techniques for neuroscience research, he subsequently accepted a position at Los Alamos National Laboratory, where he led novel technology development projects in the area of imaging. He later added an M.D., followed by residency training in diagnostic radiology at Penn State. He is currently professor and director of the Behavioral Neuroimaging Research Division in the Department of Psychiatry at Penn State College of Medicine's Hershey Medical Center and also holds additional appointments in the Department of Radiology and the Department of Neural and Behavioral Sciences. Dr. Moore has authored more than 170 scientific publications (including 66 peer-reviewed journal manuscripts), holds two U.S. patents, has won several prestigious scientific awards, is a sought-after speaker at national and international scientific meetings, and has served on numerous expert advisory committees and study sections, including the National Institutes of Health (NIH). He has received support for his research from the NIH, national foundations, and corporate sponsors. Dr. Moore's research mission is to lead the discovery, development, and validation of neuroimaging biomarkers utilizing advanced neuroimaging tools coupled with powerful bioinformatics technology to improve diagnosis, to guide pharmacologic and behavioral interventions, and to predict treatment response in children and adults devastated by brain illness. Recent developments in his laboratory include technology for rapid image-guided neurochemical and molecular interventions.

Jonathan Moreno, a member of the Institute of Medicine, is the David and Lyn Silfen University Professor and a professor of medical ethics and of history and sociology of science at the University of Pennsylvania. Dr. Moreno is also a senior fellow at the Center for American Progress in Washington, D.C. where he edits the journal *Science Progress*, and a visiting professor of biomedical ethics at the University of Virginia. His books include *Undue Risk: Secret State Experiments on Humans* (2000) and *Mind Wars: Brain Research and National Defense* (2006). He co-chaired the Committee on Guidelines for Human Embryonic Stem Cell Research, has served as a senior staff member for two presidential advisory committees, and has given invited testimony for both houses of Congress. Dr. Moreno has published more than 250 papers, reviews, and book chapters and is a member of several editorial boards. He is a frequent guest on news and information programs and is often cited and quoted in major national publications. He has served on numerous committees of the National Academies.

John R. Rasure is president and CEO of the MIND Institute, a nonprofit organization dedicated to the development of neurodiagnostic tools for brain disease and disorders. He received a Ph.D. in electrical engineering from Kansas State University. Prior to his appointment at MIND in 2005, Dr. Rasure spent over 10 years working in high tech, most recently as senior vice president at Photon Research Associates, Inc., a subsidiary of Raytheon, where he was responsible for the commercial remote sensing and geographic information systems business area and intelligence community business development related to GIS. Dr. Rasure began his career as an associate professor of electrical and computer engineering at the University of New Mexico. Within 6 years he had written more than 40 publications, secured more than $3 million in grants, and earned early promotion and tenure by building an internationally respected software research laboratory. His work focused on VLSI design, real-time image-processing architectures, visual programming, medical imaging, and remote sensing.

Mark (Danny) Rintoul is the head of the Computational Biology Department and also leads the new initiatives area for the computing sciences organization at Sandia National Laboratories. He holds a Ph.D. in computational physics from Purdue University. He is currently leading several initiatives in the laboratory related to applying state-of-the-art engineering technology and high-performance computing to problems in neural science. At Sandia, he works closely with the defense sciences organization to help integrate science and technology products into cutting-edge applications, He also serves as a liaison to the MIND Institute in Albuquerque and is an associate member of the University of New Mexico's Cancer Research and Treatment Center.

Nathan D. Schwade is the Chemical and Biological Program Manager for Threat Reduction at Los Alamos National Laboratory, where he manages a $30 million portfolio using basic and applied science to assist in threat reduction missions for national security. Dr. Schwade currently serves on several working groups for the Director of National Intelligence. He received a Ph.D. in medical sciences from Texas A&M University's Health Science Center. After a postdoctoral fellowship, Dr. Schwade accepted a faculty appointment at the University of Texas Southwestern Medical School, where he still holds an appointment as an adjunct associate professor. Dr. Schwade entered national security service in 2003 and has held several research and development management positions at Los Alamos National Laboratory. Dr. Schwade is a regular reviewer for the peer-reviewed programs for the Department of Defense and for several scholarly publications. He is also the author of 26 peer-reviewed publications and book chapters and is a regular contributor to the intelligence community.

Ronald L. Smith is in private practice of internal medicine and is an associate clinical professor at the University of Nevada School of Medicine. He was a neurobiologist at the NASA Ames Research Center and a postdoctoral fellow at the UCLA Brain Research Institute. He currently serves on the Joint Independent Science Panel on Chemical and Biological Defense and has reviewed policies, procedures, and training in troop protection from chemical, biological, and nuclear threats for the joint military services. He served on the NRC's Committee on Network Science for Future Army Applications. Dr. Smith received a Ph.D. in anatomy (neuroscience) from the University of California at San Francisco and an M.D. from the Autonomous University of Ciudad Juarez, Mexico.

Karen S. Walch is an associate professor and consultant at Thunderbird School of Global Management. She earned a Ph.D. in political science from the University of Wisconsin-Madison. She has accreditation from Harvard's Program on Negotiation; the Centre for Dispute Resolution in London; The Training Management Center, Princeton; the Hay Group, Boston; the Creativity Institute, New York; the Atwood Institute and Defensive Systems, Arizona. Dr. Walch was editor of the Conflict Resolution Series "Central America: Continuity and Change" and author of *Self-Interest and Collaboration: The CBI Experience*. She has published in *Caribbean Affairs*, the *Journal of Language of International Business*, the *Thunderbird International Business Review*, *Global Business*, the *Journal of Dispute Resolution*, and *Caribbean Choices*. She is also co-author of *Global Negotiation* and *Understanding Negotiation*. Dr. Walch currently serves as a researcher with an international team for a project on corporate cultures in global interaction, funded by the Bertelsmann Foundation, and a project on global mindset, initiated by the Garvin Center for Language and Culture.

Alice M. Young is a professor of psychology at Texas Tech University and of pharmacology and neuroscience at Texas Tech University Health Sciences Center. Her current research and teaching focus on behavioral and pharmacological processes that modulate tolerance to and dependence on psychoactive drugs, with particular attention to learning and memory processes, the roles of efficacy in psychoactive drug effects, and the roles of receptor activity in dependence and withdrawal. Before joining the Texas Tech University System in 2004, Dr. Young was a professor of psychology and of psychiatry and behavioral neurosciences at Wayne State University. Dr. Young is a past president of the Behavioral Pharmacology Society and past chair of the Division of Behavioral Pharmacology of the American Society for Pharmacology and Experimental Therapeutics. She received a Ph.D. in psychology from the University of Minnesota and post-doctoral training in pharmacology at the University of Michigan.

Appendix B

Meetings and Speakers

MEETING 1

June 19-20, 2007
The Keck Center of the National Academies
Washington, D.C.

Perspectives from the Study Sponsors
Jim Dearlove, Senior Intelligence Officer, Defense Intelligence Agency
Lily Johnston, Intelligence Community Subject Matter Expert

Cognitive and Neural Research at Walter Reed Army Institute of Research
Thomas Balkin, Chief, Department of Behavioral Biology

ONR Computational Neuroscience and Cognitive Science
Thomas McKenna, Program Officer, Office of Naval Research
Paul Bello, Office of Naval Research

Future Understanding and Analysis of Neural Function
Robert Baughman, Associate Director for Technology Development, National
    Institute of Neurological Disorders and Stroke, National Institutes of Health

Neurological Disorders and Stroke, National Institutes of Health
Walter Koroshetz, Deputy Director, Office of the Director, NINDS
Joseph Pancrazio, Lead, NINDS Neural Prosthesis Program

Methodology Briefing
Ruth David, President and CEO, ANSER, Inc. and Chair of the Technology
Insight-Gauge, Evaluate, and Review (TIGER) Standing Committee

MEETING 2

August 15-16, 2007
The Keck Center of the National Academies
Washington, D.C.

Intelligence Community Subject Matter Expert Presentation and Discussion
Lily Johnston

Intelligence Production and Utilization
Steven Thompson, Chief, Technology Warning Division, Defense Warning
Office, Defense Intelligence Agency
Rebecca Ahne, Deputy Director for Technical Intelligence, Defense Research
and Engineering
Lily Johnston

Scientific Innovation and Investment in China
Denis Simon, Provost and Chief Academic Officer, The Levin Graduate
Institute

Dynamic Decision Making in Complex Task Environments: Principles and Neural Mechanisms
Jay McClelland, Professor, Department of Psychology, Director, Center for
Mind, Brain and Computation, Stanford University

Neurotechnology Needs for Special Operations Forces
Master Chief Glenn Mercer, SOCOM SG Force Enlisted Advisor, Navy
Element SEA

Experimental Methods in Clinical Neuropsychopharmacology
Tom Kelly, Professor, Department of Behavioral Science, University of
Kentucky College of Medicine

Neural Basis of Aggressive Behavior in Cats
Allan Siegel, Professor, Department of Neurology and Neurosciences, New
Jersey Medical School

Cosmetic Neurology
Anjan Chatterjee, Associate Professor of Neurology, Center for Cognitive
    Neuroscience, University of Pennsylvania

**Trends and Developments in Neuropsychopharmacology: A 20-year
Perspective**
Jim Barrett, Senior Vice President, Chief Scientific Officer and President,
    Research, Adolor Corporation

**Combining Neuroimaging and Computational Tools to Get Real-Time
Measurements of Cognitive and Affective Processes**
Martin Paulus, Professor in Residence, Department of Psychiatry, Laboratory of
    Biological Dynamics and Theoretical Medicine, University of California,
    San Diego

**Cracking Cognition by Intergrating Single-Unity Electrophysiology, fMRI,
EEG, NIRS, and Computational Modeling**
Maximilian Riesenhuber, Assistant Professor, Laboratory for Computational
    Cognitive Neuroscience, Department of Neuroscience, Georgetown
    University Medical Center

What Functional MRI Can, Can't, and Might Not Do in The Future
Peter Bandettini, Chief, Section on Functional Imaging Methods, and Director,
    Functional MRI Core Facility, National Institutes of Health

**Optimizing Neurobehavioral Performance Through Biology and
Technology**
David Dinges, Professor of Psychology in Psychiatry and Chief of the Division
    of Sleep and Chronobiology, University of Pennsylvania School of
    Medicine

The Global Neurotechnology Industry 2007
Zack Lynch, Managing Director, Neuroinsights

**Opportunities in Cognitive/Neural Science: Assessing, Funding, and
Commercializing Innovative and Early Stage Technologies**
Mark Cochran, CEO and Executive Director, Blanchette Rockefeller
    Neurosciences Institute

MEETING 3

October 30-31, 2007
The Arnold and Mabel Beckman Center
of the National Academies
Irvine, California

Anthrocentric Multisensory Interfaces for Augmenting Cognition and Performance
Anil Raj, Research Scientist, Florida Institute for Human and Machine
    Cognition

Cognitively Plausible Software Agents
Rob Abbott, Cognitive and Exploratory Systems, Sandia National Laboratories

Immersive Virtual Environments and Psychological Processes
Jeremy Bailenson, Director, Virtual Human Interaction Laboratory, Stanford
    University

Visual Analytics: A Grand Challenge in Science—Turning Information Overload into the Opportunity of the Decade—Emphasis on Cognitive Science Needs
Jim Thomas, Director, National Visualization and Analytics Center, Pacific
    Northwest National Laboratory

Defining and Applying Cultural Anthropology
Ken Price, Vice President of Client Solutions, Training Management
    Corporation

Culture Matters
Hazel Markus, Davis-Brack Professor in the Behavioral Sciences, Co-Director
    of the Research Institute for Comparative Studies in Race and Ethnicity,
    Stanford Mind, Culture, and Society Laboratory, Stanford University

Culture, Brain, and Cognition: A Few Comments
Chuansheng Chen, Professor, Department of Psychology and Social Behavior,
    University of California, Irvine

Deception Research
Lily Johnston

Signal Detection Theory: How Bayes' Theorem Constrains Accuracy of Inference from Neurophysiologic Monitoring
Peter Imrey, Full Staff, Quantitative Health Sciences, Cleveland Clinic
 Foundation

Two Views of Brain Function
Marc Raichle, Professor of Radiology, Neurology, and Anatomy and
 Neurobiology, Mallinckrodt Institute of Radiology, Washington University
 School of Medicine

Unique Patterns of Individual Brain Activity
Mike Miller, Associate Professor of Psychology, University of California at
 Santa Barbara

MEETING 4

**January 30-31, 2008
The Arnold and Mabel Beckman Center
of the National Academies
Irvine, California**

Writing meeting.

Appendix C

Committee Methodology

With the context and scope of its assignment established, the committee turned its attention to defining a robust methodology for technology warning that would be suitable for the diverse inquiries likely to stem from ongoing engagement between a standing committee of the National Research Council (NRC) and the intelligence community's (IC's) technology warning components. The proposed methodology is described in this chapter and tested through application in subsequent chapters.

KEY FEATURES OF THE METHODOLOGY

A robust methodology for technical inquiry should have four key features. First, to be accepted, it must be presented in a lexicon and structure appropriate for the user's culture—in this case, for the culture in which the Defense Intelligence Agency (DIA) Technology Warning Division (the sponsor of this study) operates. Any communication of findings, conclusions, or recommendations offered by the committee must be expressed accordingly. The division makes use of weather-forecasting terminology (Futures, Watch, Warning, Alert)[1] in the issu-

---

NOTE: This appendix is reprinted from Avoiding Surprise in an Era of Global Technology Advances (Washington, D.C.: The National Academies Press, 2005), pp. 20-27.

[1]The definitions used by the DIA for these terms are as follows: Futures—Create a technology roadmap and forecast; identify potential observables to aid in the tracking of technological advances. Technology Watch—Monitor global communications and publications for breakthroughs and integrations. Technology Warning—Positive observables

ance of technology assessments, making the overall warning message regarding all products readily interpretable by any reader. The committee adopted and adapted the Defense Intelligence Agency (DIA)'s vocabulary to characterize the relative status—and recommended action—for each technology.

The second key feature is that, to be relevant, the study methodology must be tied in a fundamental way to top-level Department of Defense (DOD) strategies. For example, the committee reviewed Joint Vision 2020 (JCS, 2000) to validate its selection of the technology topics addressed in this report. In future studies, to facilitate integration into the larger body of intelligence materials, the committee proposes that technology selections be derived through a more disciplined, RED team[2] review of top-level strategy documents (e.g., Joint Vision 2020) with an eye to identifying technologies that could be used to deny a BLUE[3] capability deemed critical to U.S. military success.

The third key feature is that, to maintain focus and ensure timeliness, the study methodology must yield assessments built on a solid understanding of the technical feasibility of potential technology-based threats. This requirement leads to a capability-based approach for investigating and categorizing candidate technologies. Furthermore, the technical peer review process to which all NRC reports are subjected provides additional assurance of the technical quality of committee assessments.

Lastly, to be enduring, the methodology should accommodate evolving realities of science and technology (S&T) leadership, driven by the synergistic trends of globalization and commercialization described in Chapter 1. Traditionally, the United States has assumed that it leads the world in S&T. This perspective leads the technology warning community to look for indications that external actors are trying to "catch up," or to exploit known technologies in new ways. Projected trends suggest that it should no longer automatically be assumed that the United States will lead technological advances in all relevant technologies. This reality imposes a new burden on the technology warning community, generating the need for it to search in different places and in different ways for the information needed to warn against technology surprise.

---

indicate that a prototype has been achieved. Technology Alert—An adversary has been identified and operational capability is known to exist.

[2]"RED" is used in this report to denote the adversary or an adversarial perspective (e.g., "RED team").

[3]"BLUE" is used in this report to denote U.S. military forces.

FOUNDATION OF THE METHODOLOGY

The committee believes that the Technology Warning Division can most effectively prioritize its limited resources by utilizing a capabilities-based approach with respect to assessing technologies. The landscape of potentially important emerging technologies is both vast and diverse. Ideally, the division should assess whether a given technology has the potential to pose a viable threat prior to commissioning in-depth analyses. Since the division is keenly interested in when specific technologies may mature to the point that they pose a threat to U.S. forces, a functional decomposition from an adversarial, or RED, perspective is most useful. The methodology defined by the committee begins with the following focus question: *What capabilities does the United States have that, if threatened, impact U.S. military preeminence?*

In general, U.S. capabilities could be threatened either through direct denial of or disruption of BLUE capabilities or via RED capabilities that negate or significantly diminish the value of BLUE capabilities (e.g., improvised explosive devices (IEDs) being employed by insurgent forces in Iraq).

Joint Vision 2020 was used to define the basic framework for U.S. military capabilities deemed vital to sustained success (JCS, 2000). The overarching focus of this vision is Full Spectrum Dominance—achieved through the interdependent application of four operational concepts (Dominant Maneuver, Precision Engagement, Focused Logistics, and Full Dimensional Protection) and enabled through Information Superiority, as illustrated in Figure [C]-1 (JCS, 2000).

The committee selected the four operational concepts, together with Information Superiority, as the foundation for its assessment methodology. Joint Vision 2020 provides the definitions presented in Box [C]-1.

The committee also noted the importance of technology warning with respect to the "Innovation" component of Joint Vision 2020 shown in Box [C]-2, since "leaders must assess the efficacy of new ideas, the potential drawbacks to new concepts, the capabilities of potential adversaries, the costs versus benefits of new technologies, and the organizational implications of new capabilities" (JCS, 2000).

From this foundation the committee then identifies specific capabilities in accordance with the previously defined focus question—*What capabilities does the United States have that, if threatened, impact U.S. military preeminence?*

While the U.S. military has devoted significant time to the definition of vital capabilities in alignment with Joint Vision 2020, the committee made no effort in this first report to synchronize its derivations or definitions, or to provide a complete decomposition of the operational concepts and enablers into their underlying capabilities. Rather, committee

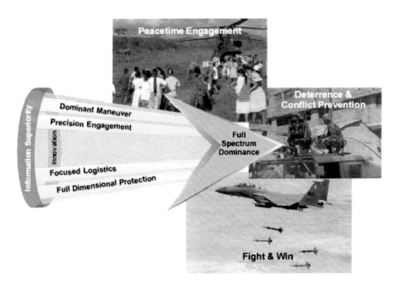

FIGURE [C]-1 Concepts constituting the basic framework for U.S. military capability as defined by Joint Vision 2020. (See Box [C]-1.) SOURCE: JCS (2000).

members selected a few evolving technologies and assessed the potential for those technologies to threaten important U.S. capabilities. Given that the committee's proposed basic methodology is adopted, future studies will analyze more comprehensively the threats to a taxonomy of U.S. military capabilities that derives from the operational concepts envisioned by Joint Vision 2020. The basic methodology developed by the committee is summarized in Box [C]-1 and is described in greater detail in subsequent sections.

IDENTIFY

The next step of the proposed assessment methodology is performed from the RED perspective. The central question here is as follows: *What are the evolving technologies that, in the hands of U.S. adversaries, might be used to threaten an important U.S. military capability?* A corollary question is, What technologies, if rapidly exploited by the U.S. military, are likely to yield sustained technological superiority? However, this issue was addressed only peripherally, given the division's focus on technology warning.

Having identified a technology of potential interest, the next challenge becomes the derivation of "indicators" or "observables" that may

BOX [C]-1
Relevant Definitions from Joint Vision 2020
Serving as Foundation for Assessment Methodology

Information Superiority is the capability to collect, process, and disseminate an uninterrupted flow of information while exploiting or denying an adversary's ability to do the same. Information superiority is achieved in a noncombat situation or one in which there are no clearly defined adversaries when friendly forces have the information necessary to achieve operational objectives.

Dominant Maneuver is the ability of joint forces to gain positional advantage with decisive speed and overwhelming operational tempo in the achievement of assigned military tasks. Widely dispersed joint air, land, sea, amphibious, special operations and space forces, capable of scaling and massing force or forces and the effects of fires as required for either combat or noncombat operations, will secure advantage across the range of military operations through the application of information, deception, engagement, mobility and counter-mobility capabilities.

Focused Logistics is the ability to provide the joint force the right personnel, equipment, and supplies in the right place, at the right time, and in the right quantity, across the full range of military operations. This will be made possible through a real-time, web-based information system providing total asset visibility as part of a common relevant operational picture, effectively linking the operator and logistician across Services and support agencies.

Precision Engagement is the ability of joint forces to locate, surveil, discern, and track objectives or targets; select, organize, and use the correct systems; generate desired effects; assess results; and reengage with decisive speed and overwhelming operational tempo as required, throughout the full range of military operations.

Full Dimensional Protection is the ability of the joint force to protect its personnel and other assets required to decisively execute assigned tasks. Full dimensional protection is achieved through the tailored selection and application of multilayered active and passive measures, within the domains of air, land, sea, space, and information across the range of military operations with an acceptable level of risk.

SOURCE: JCS (2000).

BOX [C]-2
Proposed Methodology for Technology Warning

Foundation   Joint Vision 2020 Operational Concepts and Information Superiority

- **Focus**   *What capabilities does the United States have that, if threatened, impact U.S. military preeminence?*

- **Identify**   *What are the evolving technologies that, in the hands of U.S. adversaries, might be used to threaten an important U.S. military capability?*

  What are the observables that may indicate adversarial adoption or exploitation of such technologies?

- **Assess**   *Accessibility: How difficult would it be for an adversary to exploit the technology?*

  Maturity: How much is known about an adversary's intentions to exploit the technology?

  Consequence: What is the impact on U.S. military capability should the technology be employed by an adversary?

- **Prioritize**   *Identify: What are the relative resources to be applied to each emerging technology to support the technology warning process?*

- **Task**   *Establish and assign intelligence-information-collection requirements.*

---

[a]SOURCE: JCS (2000).

---

suggest adversarial adoption or exploitation of that technology. Although targeted intelligence-collection methods remain important, in this report the committee focuses on observables that may be derived from open source analysis—leveraging the effects of the information revolution and acknowledging that the twin forces of globalization and commercialization provide new sources of relevant information. At the same time, however, the committee recognizes the difficulty of discerning when technological advances portend emerging threats rather than societal benefits.

CHART [C]-1 Example of Technology Assessment Chart

Technology		Observables
Brief description of technology		Brief description of observables
Accessibility	**Maturity**	**Consequence**
Level 1, 2, or 3	Technology Futures Technology Watch Technology Warning Technology Alert	Short characterization

A sample chart—Chart [C]-1—exemplifies how each technology is assessed.

ASSESS

The committee's assessment methodology involves characterization of a technology in terms of three variables: Accessibility, Maturity, and Consequence. Priorities for more detailed analyses may derive from any individual variable or any combination of the three.

Accessibility

The Accessibility variable focuses on the question *How difficult would it be for an adversary to exploit the technology?* It addresses the ability of an adversary to gain access to and exploit a given technology. This assessment is divided into three levels:

• *Level 1.* The technology is available through the Internet, being a commercial off-the-shelf item; low sophistication is required to exploit it.
• *Level 2.* The technology would require a small investment (hundreds to a few hundred thousand dollars) in facilities and/or expertise.
• *Level 3.* The technology would require a major investment (millions to billions of dollars) in facilities and/or expertise.

In general, Level 1 technologies are those driven by the global commercial technology environment; they are available for exploitation by a diverse range of potential adversaries. Level 3 technologies, by contrast, are typically accessible only to state-based actors. The indicators likely to be of value in determining an adversary's actual access to a given technology vary by level as well as by the type of technology.

Maturity

The Maturity variable focuses on the question *How much is known about an adversary's intentions to exploit the technology?* It integrates what is known about an adversary's actions, together with an evaluation of the state of play with respect to the technology of interest. At the highest level, called Technology Alert, an adversary has been identified and an operational capability has been observed. At the lowest level, Technology Futures, the potential for a technology-based threat has been identified, but no positive indicators have been observed. The Maturity assessment is divided into four categories: the first two (the lower levels) suggest further actions for the technology warning community; the other two indicate the need for immediate attention by military leadership:

- *Futures.* Create a technology roadmap and forecast; identify potential observables to aid in the tracking of technological advances.
- *Technology Watch.* Monitor (global) communications and publications for breakthroughs and integrations.
- *Technology Warning.* Positive observables indicate that a prototype has been achieved.
- *Technology Alert.* An adversary has been identified and operational capability is known to exist.

Given the potential for disruptive advances through technological breakthroughs or innovative integration, as well as the difficulty of identifying and tracking meaningful indicators, any particular technology is unlikely to progress sequentially through the various categories of Maturity listed above.

As indicated at the beginning of this chapter, the committee adopted and adapted the DIA's terminology in defining these categories. The definitions are likely to evolve as the process matures. The committee sees significant value in this basic approach, however, since it divorces the challenge of technology warning from the discrete time lines associated with "prediction," which are almost invariably inaccurate.

Consequence

Characterization of a technology in terms of the Consequence variable involves addressing the question *What is the impact on military capability should the technology be employed by an adversary?* It involves assessing the impact of the postulated RED technology on the capability of BLUE forces. This impact can range from denial or negation of a critical capability to the less-consequential level of annoyance or nuisance. A corollary assessment may be made as to the locus of impact—that is, whether the technology affects a single person, as in the case of an assassination, or creates a circumstance of mass casualty and attendant mass chaos.

PRIORITIZE

The objective of the prioritization step of the methodology is to respond to the question *What are the relative resources to be applied to each emerging technology to support the technology warning process?* This step is intended to harmonize the distinct nodes of observed capability, demonstrated intent, resources available, and the inherent cost of inaction. Prioritization is key to the technology warning methodology, since the Technology Warning Division lacks the resources to fully analyze every conceivable evolving technology. It is equally important to recognize that prioritization is an integral part of each methodology parameter. The prioritization of individual parameters is based on the levels of change detection and potential impact. By prioritizing the parameter, the division can focus subsequent analyses over a smaller subset of an assigned change detection domain. Priority assignment is essential to enable the focusing of more sophisticated information-gathering tools and analytic techniques on the areas of highest potential concern.

The prioritization methodology lends itself to any number of commercially available tools and techniques designed for assistance in establishing and maintaining a logical and consistent focus as well as the flexibility to react to the dynamics of technology change and country-of-interest variability. During the prioritization process, it will be important to establish measures of performance to allow critical analysis as well as change management in order to improve the overall process. The end result of the prioritization process is to provide for actionable awareness with which to influence analysis and tasking, the last of the methodology parameters.

The committee envisions that prioritization would be accomplished in close consultation with the technology warning community. It made no attempt to further develop the prioritization process in this report.

TASK

The Technology Warning Division will inevitably have unmet needs for additional information and/or intelligence relating to the prioritized list of evolving technologies. Although some needs may be met through division-chartered research, others will require the assistance of the broader intelligence community.

The task step—*Establish and assign intelligence-information-collection requirements"*—involves the dissemination of collection requirements to other IC components and subordinate agencies. Such requirements must provide sufficient specificity to enable interpretation by collectors who are not necessarily literate in the specific technology. The requirements may include general instructions for accomplishing the mission. It is envisioned that some of the observables postulated in the Identify step of the methodology will provide a useful basis for such tasking.

The results from collection efforts will be integrated back into the assessment step in order to refine, reprocess, and update the division's understanding of a given technology. This analysis may stimulate the issuance of a new report to the division's customers to inform them of changes in the assessed maturity of that technology.

USING THE METHODOLOGY IN THIS REPORT

To test the robustness of the proposed technology warning methodology, the committee applied it in order to assess four key areas in this initial report. It should be noted that this initial exercise was necessarily circumscribed by the domain expertise represented in the committee members and by the shortness of time for broader outreach to the technical community at large. Furthermore, since the methodology emerged in parallel with the committee's technology assessments, the approaches taken were not entirely consistent.

The foundation provided by Joint Vision 2020 and augmented by the military and professional backgrounds of committee members was used to select the following four key capabilities to assess:

- Information superiority (Chapter 3),
- Air superiority (Chapter 4),
- Discrimination between friends/foes/neutrals (Chapter 5), and
- Battle readiness and communications superiority (Chapter 6).

Chapters 3 through 6 each address the "Identify" activity with examples of evolving technologies that may threaten the capability and potential indicators that such technology development is under way. The "Assess" activity then examines opportunity and motivation for adversarial technology development and/or employment, posits change detection relative to the indicators, and assesses likely impact. Preliminary characterizations of accessibility, maturity, and consequence are provided for most evolving technologies, although the level of specificity is variable.

Subsequent steps (i.e., "Prioritize" and "Task") of the proposed methodology require customer inputs and actions and are left to future study efforts.

REFERENCE

JCS (Joint Chiefs of Staff). 2000. Joint Vision 2020. Director for Strategic Plans and Policy, J5; Strategy Division. U.S. Government Printing Office, Washington, D.C. June.

Appendix D

Background Information on Functional Neuroimaging

FUNCTIONAL NEAR-INFRARED SPECTROSCOPY

Principles

It is well known that the functional state of tissue can influence its optical properties (for instance, cyanosis in hypoxia and pallor in anemia). The human brain undergoes a number of physiological changes as it responds to environmental stimuli, and these changes in electrochemical activity and blood chemistry also affect the optical properties of neuronal tissues. Functional optical imaging capitalizes on those changing optical properties in measuring neural activity. Funded by the National Institutes of Health (NIH), Jöbsis (1977) and Chance et al. (1988) conducted much of the early work on brain imaging with functional near-infrared spectroscopy (fNIRS).

Neuronal activity is fueled by glucose metabolism, and increases in neural activity result in increased consumption of glucose and oxygen from the local capillary bed. A reduction in local glucose and oxygen stimulates the brain to increase local arteriolar vasodilation, which increases local cerebral blood flow (CBF) and cerebral blood volume through a mechanism known as neurovascular coupling. Over a period of several seconds, the increased CBF carries more glucose and oxygen to the area, and the oxygen is transported by oxygenated hemoglobin in the blood. The increased oxygen transported to the area typically exceeds the local rate of neuronal oxygen use, and a result is an overabundance of cerebral blood oxygenation in the active area (Fox et al., 1988). Although the initial increase in neural activity is thought to result in a focal increase in deoxygenated hemoglobin in the capillary bed as oxygen is withdrawn from the hemoglobin for use in the metabolism of glucose, this part of the vascular response has been much more difficult to measure, and more controversial, than hyperoxygenation. (See Buxton, 2001 and Obrig et al., 1996, 2000a,b, for more detailed discussion of this topic.)

Because oxygenated and deoxygenated hemoglobin (oxy-Hb and deoxy-Hb) have characteristic optical properties in the visible and near-infrared light range, the change in their concentrations during neurovascular coupling can be measured optically (Chance et al., 1998; Villringer and Chance, 1997). Most biological tissues are relatively transparent to light in the near-infrared range of 700-900 nm largely because water absorption is relatively low at these wavelengths. However, the chromophores oxy-Hb and deoxy-Hb absorb specific wavelengths in that range. Thus, that spectral band is often referred to as the optical window for the noninvasive assessment of brain activation (Jöbsis, 1977). Photons introduced at the scalp pass through most of the tissue and are either scattered by it or absorbed by oxy-Hb and deoxy-Hb. Because a relatively predictable quantity of photons follows a banana-shaped path back to the surface of the skin, the photons can be measured at the scalp with photodetectors (Gratton et al., 1994). Changes in the chromophore concentrations cause changes in the intensity of detected light and are quantified according to a modified Beer-Lambert law, essentially an empirical description of optical attenuation in a highly scattering medium (Cope and Delpy, 1988; Cope, 1991). If absorbance changes at two (or more) wavelengths, one of which is more sensitive to oxy-Hb and another to deoxy-Hb, are measured, changes in the relative concentrations of these chromophores can be calculated. Using those principles, researchers have demonstrated that it is possible to assess brain activity through the intact skull in adult humans (Chance et al., 1993; Gratton et al., 1995; Hoshi and Tamura, 1993; Kato et al., 1993; Villringer et al., 1993). Other chromophores, including cytochrome-c oxidase, can also be assessed optically. Cytochrome-c oxidase, a marker of metabolic demands, holds the potential to provide more direct information about neuronal activity than hemoglobin (Heekeren et al., 1999; Jöbsis, 1977). However, because cytochrome-c oxidase is used much less often than the hemoglobin-based measures, it will not be discussed further here (see Heekeren et al. [1999] for more detail).

Typically, an fNIRS apparatus comprises a light source, which is coupled to the participant's head via either light-emitting diodes (LEDs) or fiber-optic bundles, and a light detector that receives light after it has interacted with tissue. Light scatters after entering tissue, and a photodetector placed 2-7 cm away from the optode, an optical sensor device that optically measures a specific substance usually with the aid of a chemical transducer, can collect light after it has passed through tissue. When the distance between the source and the photodetector is set at 4 cm, the fNIRS signal is sensitive to hemodynamic changes within the top 2-3 mm of the cortex and extends 1 cm to either side perpendicular to the source-detector axis (Chance et al., 1988). Studies have shown that the gray matter of the cortex can be imaged with interoptode distances as short as 2 cm (Chance et al., 1988; Firbank et al., 1998). Several types of brain activity have been assessed with this technique, including motor activity, visual activation, auditory stimulation, and performance of cognitive tasks (e.g., Villringer and Chance, 1997).

Fast Functional Near-Infrared Spectroscopy

A second, more controversial method, called the event-related optical signal (EROS), capitalizes on changes in the optical properties of cell membranes that occur when a neuron "fires," or is activated (Gratton et al., 1995). When a neuron is activated, ionic fluxes across the cell membrane (such as shifts in sodium and potassium ions) result in a change in the membrane potential. The ionic fluxes also change the magnetic and electrical fields around the neuron, which, when summed across a large number of synchronously activated neurons, constitute the signal that is assessed with electroencephalography (EEG) or magnetoencephalography (MEG). By using invasive techniques, it has been established that the optical properties of neural membranes differ between the depolarized state and the resting state (Obrig and Villringer, 2003; Rector et al., 1997; Stepnoski et al., 1991) and that optical methods can be used to detect the differences.

There are a number of limitations of the noninvasive use of EROS in humans. A primary disadvantage of the fast optical signal is the high signal-to-noise ratio that results from the need to image through skin, skull, and cerebrospinal fluid. Basic sensory and motor activities, such as tactile stimulation and finger-tapping, require 500-1000 trials to establish a reliable signal (Franceschini and Boas, 2004). There have been failures in attempting to replicate the results of experiments that reported the EROS in response to a visual stimulus in healthy adult humans (Syre et al., 2004). Final constraints are that these methods require a more expensive and cumbersome laser-based light source (as opposed to an LED-based light source), they are not portable, and there is a greater risk of inadvertent damage to the eyes than with the systems available for measuring hemodynamic responses; LED-based near-infrared sources pose very little, if any, risk to the eyes (Bozkurt and Onaral, 2004).

Despite current limitations, the fast optical signal continues to be an important subject of investigation because it offers glimpses of the "holy grail" of neuroimaging: the direct measurement of neuronal activity with millisecond resolution and superior spatial resolution. The potential for implanted optodes is particularly important. Because the optical signal can be carried by fiber optics, implanted optodes would allow extremely precise localization of neural activity, in addition to millisecond resolution. Proximity to the tissue would greatly reduce the amount of light power required for imaging and thus lower both the power consumption and the heat output of the optodes. Optodes used to image the cortex could be implanted just below the surface of the skull, allowing the cerebrospinal fluid to remain as a buffer and thereby avoiding the scarring that interferes with chronically implanted EEG electrodes. Fiber optics might have some of the same problems as implanted EEG electrodes for deep tissue (such as scar-tissue buildup), but as some of the problems yield to advancing research, fNIRS optodes could potentially be implanted for deep-tissue assessment. At least one U.S. grant has been issued to investigate the feasibility of implanted fNIRS optodes in animals.

Current applications include the restoration of mobility in hemiplegic and paraplegic patients. For example, brain-computer interfaces could potentially be driven by signals in the motor cortex. The same brain-computer interfaces could potentially be used in military applications, such as weapons control (Peters et al, 2008). Overall system cost will be relatively low in a few years, and the rate-limiting factor in the near future may be the cost of surgery.

Functional Near-Infrared Spectroscopy Systems

A wide variety of commercial and custom-built fNIRS instruments are in use (Strangman et al., 2002). The systems differ with respect to their use and engineering, specifically among light sources, detectors, and instrument electronics. Three distinct types of fNIRS implementation have been developed: time-resolved systems, frequency-domain systems, and continuous-wave (CW) spectroscopy; each has its own strengths and limitations. CW spectroscopy applies continuous or slow-pulse (up to several kilohertz) light to tissue and measures the attenuation of amplitude of the incident light (Strangman et al., 2002; Hoshi, 2003; Izzetoglu et al., 2004; Obrig and Villringer, 2003). CW systems provide somewhat less information than time-resolved or frequency-domain systems, but they have several advantages for some applications: they can be manufactured far less expensively than time-resolved and frequency-domain systems, and they can be very small, so they are practical for use in clinical and educational settings. Laser-based time-resolved or frequency-domain systems provide information on both phase and amplitude and allow more precise quantification of fNIRS signals. (For more discussion of system differences, see Boas et al., 2002; Hoshi, 2003; Izzetoglu et al., 2004; Obrig and Villringer, 2003; and Strangman et al., 2002.)

Comparison of Functional Near-Infrared Spectroscopy with Other Neuroimaging Modalities

Early efforts to develop neurobiological models of cognition and emotion relied on EEG or event-related potential (ERP), which are measures of physiological function. Those measures have several advantages for research. They are relatively inexpensive, are noninvasive, and have nearly instantaneous time resolution. They can be used with infants and children, as well as adults, and can be used repeatedly with no adverse effects. As a result, applications of EEG and ERP have contributed important data for developing models of cognitive and emotional processing. However, EEG measures are limited in their ability to provide the precise location of an electrical source. EEG does yield spatial information, but it must be reconstructed with probabilistic models. Although mathematical models are improving, EEG, even when applied in very-high-density fields, can provide only a relative approximation of current sources.

The introduction of neuroimaging modalities, such as functional magnetic resonance imaging (fMRI) and positron-emission tomography, has made it possible to examine much more precisely the anatomical location of the neural circuitry underlying various mental events in humans. Many clinicians are familiar with the basic principles of fMRI and use the results of fMRI research to inform their clinical practice and research. fMRI is considered the "gold standard" for measuring functional brain activation because it offers safe, noninvasive neuroimaging with high spatial resolution. It is therefore useful to compare fNIRS with the well-known technology of fMRI (see Gore, 2003, for a clear and more comprehensive description of the principles of fMRI). The primary measure used for fMRI is the blood-oxygen-level–dependent (BOLD) signal that accompanies neuronal activation in the brain and is secondary, for instance, to the presentation of a stimulus. As previously discussed, increase in CBF to an active area exceeds the additional neuronal metabolic demand and results in a decrease in deoxy-Hb concentration in the local tissue. The magnetic susceptibility of blood containing oxy-Hb differs very little from that of water or other tissues that have low paramagnetic properties. However, deoxy-Hb is highly paramagnetic and therefore has very different magnetic properties from surrounding tissues and can act as a naturally occurring contrast agent (Pauling and Coryell, 1936). The presence of deoxygenated blood in a given area results in a less uniform magnetic field. Because the magnetic resonance signal depends on the uniformity of the magnetic field experienced by water molecules, less uniformity (that is, when more deoxy-Hb is present) results in less signal clarity and in more rapid decay of the overall signal. In contrast, as the deoxygenated blood in a given area is replaced with oxygenated blood, the local magnetic environment becomes more uniform, and the MRI signal lasts longer and is therefore stronger during image acquisition. The signal change is typically around 1 percent or less, depending on the strength of the magnetic field. Therefore, fMRI, like fNIRS, is an indirect measure of neuronal activity that assesses changes in the concentration of deoxy-Hb in local tissue. There is no simple relationship between the magnitude of the signal change and any single physiological measure inasmuch as the magnitude relies on changes in blood flow, blood volume, and local oxygen tension. There is also a delay between the time when the local neurons are activated and begin to use oxygen and the time when vasodilation occurs and allows increased blood flow and the transport of oxy-Hb to the area. The latter process, called the hemodynamic response, occurs over several seconds after the initiation of neuronal activity.

The more commonly used fNIRS technology (use of the measurement of hemoglobin-based chromophores) has much in common with the BOLD-based signal in that it measures relative changes in concentrations of deoxy-Hb that depend on the hemodynamic response. Both are indirect measures of neural activity, with temporal resolution measured in seconds, because they are limited by the hemodynamic response. Both provide spatial resolution, are safe, are noninvasive, and can be used repeatedly in the same people. Because of their signal-to-noise ratios, both technologies typically require repeated stimulation.

There are also, however, important differences between the two technologies. fNIRS is unlikely to supplant fMRI in basic research on the neurophysiological underpinnings of various cognitive, emotional, and motivational processes, for two important reasons. First, fMRI has better spatial resolution, around 1 mm^2, although the fast imaging of fMRI reduces its spatial resolution somewhat (to a few millimeters) relative to conventional MRI. In contrast, because of the scatter of photons in a diverse medium, current fNIRS systems have a spatial resolution of around 1 cm^2. Second, fMRI has the capacity to image the entire brain, whereas fNIRS is limited to the outer cortex. Although a large hemorrhage might be able to be imaged as deep as the thalamus with fNIRS, more subtle signals, such as those induced by a cognitive or emotional event, are limited to a depth of about 2-4 mm of the cortex.

fNIRS has a number of advantageous properties that hold enormous potential for research studies and clinical applications that require the quantitative measurement of hemodynamic changes in the cortex under a variety of conditions not amenable to fMRI. The limitations of fMRI relative to fNIRS include the need for subjects to lie within the confines of the magnet bore and the refrigerant systems used to supercool the magnets also produce loud noises that can interfere with some protocols. fMRI is also highly sensitive to movement; subjects' movements of a few millimeters can invalidate the data. The intense strength of the magnets necessary to create the MRI signal precludes the use of any ferrous metals in or around the magnet. Finally, fMRI systems are expensive—an initial cost of a few million dollars, depending on the strength of the magnet—and individual participant runs can cost several hundred dollars each.

FUNCTIONAL SPECIALIZATION

The human brain evolved in layers, with evolutionarily newer structures covering older ones. The developing brain in a human embryo grows outward in a pattern that largely mirrors human evolution. The brain is divided into discrete regions that control vital functions, such as sensory transduction and cognition in the case of the cortex. Such functional specialization is a critical element in brain research, and it arises mainly from layered development. The functionally specific regions "activate" when a person is presented with a stimulus or task; for example, smells excite an area of the temporal lobe, and vision excites the occipital lobe.

Mapping the areas of activation and the circuits that control specific behaviors and cognitive processes is the goal of functional neuroimaging. It is an enormous goal in light of the relative size of the target, and creating even a crude map of the functionality of the brain is daunting. The brain involves many more connections than the most advanced computer because, unlike a computer that uses binary connections, brain circuits involve thousands of neurons and millions of connections in performing even the simplest task of cognition or behavior. Indeed, one can think of gray matter neurons as transistors and white matter fibers as the wires that connect the transistors, although in the brain each neuron can have multiple connections—even 10,000 or more.

To provide some perspective on the enormity of the task of mapping connected areas, a typical human infant has about 1 billion gray matter neurons. With the exception of some interesting findings that suggest continuing neurogenesis in the dentate gyrus (a portion of the midbrain), the newborn will never grow any more neurons. If almost no new neurons are developing, from where does all the extra mass come? Although the number of neurons is largely fixed at birth, the brain continually forms complex white matter connections between neurons at an almost inconceivable rate. The human infant may form 20,000 distinct neural connections every second for the first year of life. Those are merely individual connections. If we factor in circuits that involve thousands or tens of thousands or even millions of reciprocal connections,[1] it becomes clear that there are far more combinations of neural circuits in the cerebral cortex than atoms in the known universe.[2]

Cautious but undaunted, scientists are busily mapping the connectivity of the human brain in thousands of new papers published each year. Many studies are investigating correlations between traditional psychological testing, clinical observations, and brain scans to establish biomarkers of pathological states, cognitive and behavioral tasks, task-specific aptitude measures, detection of deception, and even prediction of neuropathological propensity.

REFERENCES

Boas, D., J. Culver, J. Stott, and A. Dunn. 2002. Three dimensional Monte Carlo code for photon migration through complex heterogeneous media including the adult human head. *Optics Express* 10(3):159-170.

Bozkurt, A., and B. Onaral. 2004. Safety assessment of near infrared light emitting diodes for diffuse optical measurements. *BioMedical Engineering OnLine* 3(1):9. Available from http://www.biomedical-engineering-online.com/content/3/1/9. Last accessed February 13, 2008.

Buxton, R.B. 2001. The elusive initial dip. *NeuroImage* 13(6):953-958.

Chance B., E. Anday, S. Nioka, S. Zhou, S. Long, K. Worden, C. Li, T. Murray, Y. Ovetsky, D. Pidikiti, and R. Thomas. 1998. A novel method for fast imaging of brain function, non-invasively, with light. *Optics Express* 2(10):411-423.

---

[1]For example, if there are 1,000 possible combinations in the first link of a neural circuit, the number of combinations with a second reciprocal link would be $1,000 \times 999 \times 998$ all the way down to 1, or 1000!, which is about 10^{2568}.

[2]There are around 10^{80} atoms in the visible universe and perhaps 10^{82} if we include nonluminous matter. For additional information, see http://www.holisticeducator.com. Accessed January 24, 2008.

Chance, B., J.S. Leigh, H. Miyake, D.S. Smith, S. Nioka, R. Greenfeld, M. Finander, K. Kaufmann, W. Levy, M. Young, P. Cohen, H. Yoshioka, and R. Boretsky. 1988. Comparison of time-resolved and -unresolved measurements of deoxyhemoglobin in brain. *Proceedings of the National Academy of Sciences U.S.A.* 85(14):4971-4975.

Chance, B., Z. Zhuang, C. UnAh, C. Alter, and L. Lipton. 1993. Cognition-activated low-frequency modulation of light absorption in human brain. *Proceedings of the National Academy of Sciences U.S.A.* 90(8):3770-3774.

Cope M. 1991. The development of a near infrared spectroscopy system and its application for non invasive monitoring of cerebral blood and tissue oxygenation in the newborn infant. Ph.D. thesis, University College London.

Cope, M., and D.T. Delpy. 1988. System for long-term measurement of cerebral blood and tissue oxygenation on newborn infants by near infra-red transillumination. *Medical and Biological Engineering and Computing* 26(3):289-294.

Firbank, M., E. Okada, and D.T. Delpy. 1998. A theoretical study of the signal contribution of regions of the adult head to near-infrared spectroscopy studies of visual evoked responses. *NeuroImage* 8(1):69-78.

Fox, P.T., M.E. Raichle, M.A. Mintun, and C. Dence. 1988. Nonoxidative glucose consumption during focal physiologic neural activity. *Science* 241(4864):462-464.

Franceschini, M., and D.A. Boas. 2004. Noninvasive measurement of neuronal activity with near-infrared optical imaging. *NeuroImage* 21(1):372-386.

Gore, John C. 2003. Principles and practice of functional MRI of the human brain. *Journal of Clinical Investigation* 112(1):4-9.

Gratton, G., J.S. Maier, M. Fabiani, W.W. Mantulin, and E. Gratton. 1994. Feasibility of intracranial near-infrared optical scanning. *Psychophysiology* 31(2):211-215.

Gratton, G., M. Fabiani, D. Friedman, M.A. Franceschini, S. Fantini, P.M. Corballis, and E. Gratton. 1995. Rapid changes of optical parameters in the human brain during a tapping task. *Journal of Cognitive Neuroscience* 7(4):446-456.

Heekeren, H.R., M. Kohl, H. Obrig, R. Wenzel, W. Von Pannwitz, S.J. Matcher, U. Dirnagl, C.E. Cooper, and A. Villringer. 1999. Noninvasive assessment of changes in cytochrome-c oxidase oxidation in human subjects during visual stimulation. *Journal of Cerebral Blood Flow and Metabolism* 19(6):592-603.

Hoshi, Y. 2003. Functional near-infrared optical imaging: utility and limitations in human brain mapping. *Psychophysiology* 40(4):511-520.

Hoshi, Y., and M. Tamura. 1993. Dynamic multichannel near-infrared optical imaging of human brain activity. *Journal of Applied Physiology* 75(4):1842-1846.

Izzetoglu, K., S. Bunce, M. Izzetoglu, B. Onaral, K. 2004. Functional near-infrared neuroimaging. Invited Paper, Symposium on Recent Advances in Neural Engineering. Pp. 5333-5336 in *Proceedings of the 26th Annual International Conference of the IEEEE EMBS*. San Francisco, CA, September 1-5, 2004.

Jöbsis, F.F. 1977. Noninvasive, infrared monitoring of cerebral and myocardial oxygen sufficiency and circulatory parameters. *Science* 198(4323):1264-1267.

Kato, T., A. Kamei, S. Takashima, and T. Ozaki. 1993. Human visual cortical function during photic stimulation monitoring by means of near-infrared spectroscopy. *Journal of Cerebral Blood Flow and Metabolism* 13:516-520.

Obrig H., and A. Villringer. 2003. Beyond the visible—imaging the human brain with light. *Journal of Cerebral Blood Flow and Metabolism* 23(1):1-18.

Obrig, H., C. Hirth, J.G. Junge-Hulsing, C. Doge, T. Wolf, U. Dirnagl, and A. Villringer. 1996. Cerebral oxygenation changes in response to motor stimulation. *Journal of Applied Physiology* 81(3):1174-1183.

Obrig H., M. Neufang, R. Wenzel, M. Kohl, J. Steinbrink, K. Einhaupl, and A.Villringer. 2000a. Spontaneous low frequency oscillations of cerebral hemodynamics and metabolism in human adults. *NeuroImage* 12(6):623-639.

Obrig H., R. Wenzel, M. Kohl, S. Horst, P. Wobst, J. Steinbrink, F. Thomas, and A. Villringer. 2000b. Near-infrared spectroscopy: Does it function in functional activation studies of the adult brain? *International Journal of Psychophysiology* 35(2):125-142.

Pauling, L., and C.D. Coryell. 1936. The magnetic properties and structure of hemoglobin, oxyhemoglobin and carbonmonoxy-hemoglobin. *Proceedings of the National Academy of Sciences U.S.A.* 22(4):210-216.

Peters, David, Richard Genik, and Christopher Green. 2008. Neuroimaging in defense policy. Pp. 1-42 in *Biotechnology and the Future of America's Military: The "New" Biological Warfare*. Washington, DC: National Defense University Press, in press.

Rector, D.M., G.R. Poe, M.P. Kristensen, and R.M. Harper. 1997. Light scattering changes follow evoked potentials from hippocampal Schaeffer collateral stimulation. *Journal of Neurophysiology* 78(3):1707-1713.

Stepnoski R.A., A. LaPorta, F. Raccuia-Behling, G.E. Blonder, R.E. Slusher, and D. Kleinfeld. 1991. Noninvasive detection of changes in membrane potential in cultured neurons by light scattering. *Proceedings of the National Academy of Sciences U.S.A.* 88(21):9382-9386.

Strangman, G., J.P. Culver, J.H. Thompson, and D.A. Boas. 2002. A quantitative comparison of simultaneous BOLD fMRI and NIRS recordings during functional brain activation. *NeuroImage* 17(2):719-731.

Syre, F., H. Obrig, J. Steinbrink, M. Kohl, R. Wenzel, and A. Villringer. 2004. Are VEP correlated fast optical signals detectable in the human adult by non-invasive near infrared spectroscopy (NIRS)? *Advances in Experimental Medicine and Biology* 530:421-431.

Villringer, A., and B. Chance. 1997. Non-invasive optical spectroscopy and imaging of human brain function. *Trends in Neurosciences* 20(10):435-442.

Villringer, A., J. Planck, C. Hock, L. Schleinkofer, and U. Dirnagl. 1993. Near infrared spectroscopy (NIRS): A new tool to study hemodynamic changes during activation of brain function in human adults. *Neuroscience Letters* 154(1-2):101-104.

Appendix E

Background Information on Neuroethics

The most recent authoritative document on research ethics is the *International Ethical Guidelines for Biomedical Research Involving Human Subjects*, issued by the Council for International Organizations of Medical Sciences (CIOMS) in 1993 and revised in 2002 (Council for International Organizations of Medical Sciences, 2002). CIOMS is an international, nongovernment, nonprofit organization established jointly by the World Health Organization[1] (WHO) and the UN Educational, Scientific and Cultural Organization (UNESCO)[2] in 1949. The CIOMS guidelines are based on the stipulation that all research involving human subjects should be conducted in accordance with three basic ethical principles: respect for persons, beneficence, and justice. It is generally agreed that those principles, which in the abstract have equal moral force, guide the conscientious preparation of proposals for scientific studies. The CIOMS guidelines are directed at the practical application of the three principles to human-subjects research.

The 1993 CIOMS guidelines provided a concise and clear overview of the existing ethical guidance for human-subjects research (Council for International Organizations of Medical Sciences, 2002):

> The first international instrument on the ethics of medical research, the Nuremberg Code, was promulgated in 1947 as a consequence of the trial of physicians (the Doctors' Trial) who had conducted atrocious experiments on

---

[1]For additional information, see WHO's Web site, http://www.who.int. Accessed on December 20, 2007.

[2]For additional information, see UNESCO's Web site, http://www.unesco.org. Accessed on December 20, 2007.

unconsenting prisoners and detainees during the second world war. The Code, designed to protect the integrity of the research subject, set out conditions for the ethical conduct of research involving human subjects, emphasizing their voluntary consent to research.

The Universal Declaration of Human Rights was adopted by the General Assembly of the United Nations in 1948. To give the Declaration legal as well as moral force, the General Assembly adopted in 1966 the International Covenant on Civil and Political Rights. Article 7 of the Covenant states *"No one shall be subjected to torture or to cruel, inhuman or degrading treatment or punishment. In particular, no one shall be subjected without his free consent to medical or scientific experimentation".* It is through this statement that society expresses the fundamental human value that is held to govern all research involving human subjects—the protection of the rights and welfare of all human subjects of scientific experimentation.

The Declaration of Helsinki, issued by the World Medical Association in 1964, is the fundamental document in the field of ethics in biomedical research and has influenced the formulation of international, regional and national legislation and codes of conduct. The Declaration, amended several times, most recently in 2000 . . ., is a comprehensive international statement of the ethics of research involving human subjects. It sets out ethical guidelines for physicians engaged in both clinical and nonclinical biomedical research.

Since the first publication of the CIOMS 1993 Guidelines, several international organizations have issued ethical guidance on clinical trials. This has included, from the World Health Organization, in 1995, *Guidelines for Good Clinical Practice for Trials on Pharmaceutical Products*; and from the International Conference on Harmonisation of Technical Requirements for Registration of Pharmaceuticals for Human Use (ICH),[3] in 1996, *Guideline on Good Clinical Practice*, designed to ensure that data generated from clinical trials are mutually acceptable to regulatory authorities in the European Union, Japan and the United States of America.

In his 2005 article, John Williams, member of the Ethics Unit of the World Medical Association, laid out exactly on which points the documents essentially are in agreement (Williams, 2005):

> Despite the different scope, length, and authorship of these documents, they agree to a very large extent on the basic requirements of research ethics, namely:
>
> • every proposal for medical research on human subjects must be reviewed and approved by an independent ethics committee before it can proceed;
> • a medical research project involving human subjects must be justifiable on scientific grounds;

---

[3]For additional information, see ICH's Web site, http://www.ich.org. Accessed on December 20, 2007.

- a medical research project must contribute to the well-being of society in general;
- the risks to the research subjects must not be unreasonable or disproportionate to the expected benefits of the research;
- research on human subjects cannot proceed without their informed consent;
- research subjects have a right to privacy with regard to their personal health information;
- research results must be reported accurately;
- anyone who has knowledge of unethical research has an obligation to disclose this information to the appropriate authorities.

Not specifically concerned with biomedical research involving human subjects but clearly pertinent, as noted above, are international human-rights instruments, mainly the Universal Declaration of Human Rights (United Nations, 1948), which, particularly in its science provisions, was highly influenced by the Nuremberg Code;[4] the International Covenant on Civil and Political Rights (United Nations, 1966a);[5] and the International Covenant on Economic, Social and Cultural Rights (United Nations, 1966b). Since the Nuremberg experience, human-rights law has expanded to include the protection of women (Convention on the Elimination of All Forms of Discrimination Against Women, United Nations, 1979) and children (Convention on the Rights of the Child, United Nations, 1989). Those and other such international instruments endorse, in terms of human rights, the general ethical principles that underlie such documents as the CIOMS *International Ethical Guidelines.*

Principles guiding the ethical treatment of human research subjects have been incorporated into the laws or regulations of many countries and international organizations, including those which deal with the approval of drugs and medical devices. Not all aspects of research ethics enjoy general agreement. As medical science continues to advance in, for example, genetics, the neurosciences, and organ and tissue regeneration, questions arise regarding the ethical acceptability of new techniques, procedures, and treatments for which there are no ready-made answers.

The source of one of the most well-known documents guiding human-subjects research, the Declaration of Helsinki (DoH), The World Medical Association (WMA) (1964)[6] is the global federation of national medical associations representing millions of physicians worldwide. Acting on behalf of patients and physicians, WMA endeavors to achieve the highest possible standards of medi-

---

[4]*Trials of War Criminals before the Nuremberg Military Tribunals under Control Council Law No. 10,* Vol. 2, pp. 181-182. Washington, D.C.: U.S. Government Printing Office, 1949.

[5]For additional information, see the UN Office of the High Commissioner for Human Rights Web site, http://www.ohchr.org/EN/Pages/WelcomePage.aspx. Accessed on March 28, 2008.

[6]For additional information, see WMA's Web site at http://www.wma.net. Accessed on December 20, 2007.

cal care, ethics, education, and health-related human rights for all people. Otmar Kloiber, WMA secretary general, reported on inquiry[7,8] that:

> the World Medical Association entrusts it completely to its members to implement and monitor the implementation of WMA policy. The office of the WMA has neither the means nor the task to investigate the application in the countries. With the Declaration of Helsinki the implementation has been fairly successful but yet we don't have reliable country data. For a country such as Iran we simply don't know.

That implies that although the DoH has international authority, it is not known how well it is respected or even enforced across the globe. Dr. Kloiber continued: "A very strong role lies in the hand of the publishers of international professional journals. Requirements to give proof of the observation of the DoH certainly help to get those standards accepted."

That last remark shows that overt research that is submitted for publication to (ideally) peer-reviewed professional journals must meet the highest standards of human research-subject protection as exemplified by the DoH and the CIOMS guidelines. Covert or classified military research findings will probably *not* be submitted for publication in the international literature, so they will escape the attention of publishers and peer reviewers. Thus, human-subjects protection in this sector of biomedical research cannot be guaranteed or assessed. Military use of advances in biomedical science is extremely difficult to investigate, because of the classified status of most such research. To safeguard their national security, nations that are actively pursuing biotechnology useful to the military are highly unlikely to advertise their accomplishments in the biomedical literature or elsewhere. Moreover, an inverse relationship seems apparent: countries that are most likely to be pursuing neuroscientific and other biotechnological developments for military or intelligence use are least likely to be direct or transparent about such activities.

The international community is concerned about the reactivation of the nuclear program in Iran. The recent visit of the Iranian president to the UN in New York has not relieved any of the fears associated with Iran's development of nuclear power (Hoge, 2007). And the development of other forms of military technologies, such as neurotechnological devices, to build Iran's national defense and perhaps even offense remains largely unknown. It poses a threat to international stability, and we are compelled to learn more about ethical regulations for biomedical research in Iran.

---

[7]For this report, representatives of WMA, CIOMS, and the International Association for Bioethics were approached with specific questions about the scope of and international compliance with their guidelines. Only WMA responded to the committee's request.

[8]Otmar Kloiber, WMA, personal communication to committee member Jonathan Moreno on September 18, 2007.

Bioethics in Iran is largely influenced by the Islamic underpinnings of its society but reportedly takes international documents and guidelines into account. In a 2007 article, Iranian physicians Larijani and Zahedi give an extensive overview of the status of medical ethics in their country (Larijani and Zahedi, 2007):

> Establishment of Medical Ethics Research Center by Ministry of Health and Medical education (MOHME) in 1993, formation of Medical Ethics Research Committees at National level (1997), formation of Medical Ethics Research Committees at University level for monitoring research, implementation of the National Code for ethics in Biomedical Research all over the country, and translating and authoring books on medical ethics and ethics in research have been the early activities in Iran. "Medical Ethics with a Brief Overview of Medical History" (1991) is one of the reference books for medical students in Iran which was published by MOHME in collaboration with the faculties of the Tehran University of Medical Sciences.
>
> The First International Conference on Medical Ethics (Tehran, 1993), seminars and short-courses on medical ethics for physicians, nurses and pharmacists, weekly workshops on research ethics for medical researchers in different regions of the country are being conducted.
>
> The National Codes of Ethics for biomedical research (26 codes) was prepared by MOHME in 2000. These codes are in accordance with the international declarations such as Helsinki Declaration and have been customized according to Islamic codes and Iranian cultural issues.
>
> Consequently, the Specific National Ethical Guidelines for Biomedical Research were compiled in 2005. The primary draft has been reviewed by some law, ethics, medical and religious experts. The guidelines contain "Ethical Guidelines for Clinical Trials", "Ethical Guidelines for Research on Vulnerable Groups", "Ethical Guidelines for Genetic Research", "Ethical Guidelines for Gamete and Embryo Research", "Ethical Guidelines for Transplantation Research", and "Ethical Guidelines for Research on Animals". The Guidelines have been ratified and forwarded to the universities and research centers in spring 2006.

The concept of human dignity is rooted firmly in Islam, and respect for human participants in biomedical research should follow directly from it. In addition, Iran is a member state of the UN and has confirmed its adherence to UN and UNESCO documents on human rights. However, the Iranian record of questionable treatment of (assumed) homosexuals, women, and secular scholars does not bolster confidence that both international and Iranian bioethics guidelines will always be complied with by Iranian government biomedical researchers.

Iran has a strong tradition of scientific inquiry and scholarly activities. Universities foster national and international scientific collaboration and exchange of ideas, as exemplified by a recent international conference on biotechnology. The conference was organized by the National Institute for Genetic Engineering and

Biotechnology in Tehran; the Asian and Pacific Centre for Transfer of Technology in New Delhi, India; and the Korea Research Institute for Bioscience and Biotechnology in Daejeon, Korea. During a presentation about the development of expertise in nanobiotechnology, Mohsen Jahanshahi, of the University of Mazandaran in Iran, discussed the neuroscientific uses of nanotechnology in Iran (Jahanshahi, 2005). Specifically, techniques for monitoring human performance, brain-machine interfaces, modulation of brain structure, and artificial brains with natural intelligence were mentioned. That shows that at least at one center in Iran with expertise in neuroscience is being developed, although not specifically for military use. It is easy to find information on biotechnology, with respect to both the research setting and biotechnology companies, on Iranian Web sites, but it is not at all straightforward to find out how much of the research is connected to cognitive neuroscience and possible advances in science related to national defense.

China is fast becoming an international superpower and a haven for biotechnology research. Relatively inexpensive labor and the presence of biotechnological expertise in universities and companies make China an attractive location for international biomedical research. China seems to have been taking steps in recent years to increase transparency and accountability in biomedical research (Jia, 2006). In May 2007, Qiu Renzong, honorary director of the Centre for Applied Ethics at the Chinese Academy of Social Sciences in Beijing, wrote in a Web publication about the proposed new ethics regulations to govern biomedical research (Renzong, 2007):

> Until recently, there has been little control of ethical review in these sectors [biomedical research]. In January this year—following around nine years of debate among Chinese scientists, bioethicists and policymakers—China's Ministry of Health finally approved the country's first general regulations on ethical review of biomedical research involving human subjects.

Renzong goes on to state:

> The new Chinese regulations successfully fit ethical review within the country's own laws and regulations while also abiding by international bioethical principles. They clearly state that the process of ethical review should be independent, objective, just and transparent.
>
> The regulations encompass a three-tier infrastructure made up of national, provincial and institutional ethical committees. They outline the wider principles of ethical review, the requirements for obtaining informed consent or establishing a research protocol, and the penalties that will be applied for violating the rules. The new regulations prioritise individuals' health and safety over scientific and societal interests.

However, implementation of the new regulations is not final, as Renzong explains:

> But drafting the regulation is only the first step in making human subject protection sustainable. Implementing it, and ensuring its widespread adoption will be a far more demanding and formidable task—but one that, if successful, will give much-needed impetus to building Chinese capacity in research ethics.
>
> Much should—and is—being done to help China succeed. The Ministry for Health's ethics committee is busy drafting key documents such as the constitutions of the proposed ethics committees and application forms for principal investigators to use when seeking ethical approval that can be used nationwide. Existing institutional ethics committees are also being monitored by the ministry and provincial healthcare administrations to assess how and if they work, and to consider where they need re-organising or re-establishing.
>
> Great efforts are also being made to train researchers, ethics committee members and healthcare administrators responsible for governing ethical review.
>
> National and foreign institutes—including the Peking Union Medical College, Huazhong University of Science and Technology and Fudan University in China and the US-based universities of Harvard, California, Chicago and Yale, among others—have been collaborating since 2004 to provide such training. They have organised research ethics workshops for Chinese stakeholders across the country.

Those are promising, yet early, developments in the protection and safety of human participants of biomedical research, especially in a country that has a questionable record of abuse of prisoners for medical purposes, such as organ transplantation. It should also be noted that the formal document with the bioethics regulations discussed by Renzong was not available at the official Web site of the Chinese government as of September 2007.

Humane treatment of military personnel as human research subjects is still not readily assessable, although there seems to be some transparency in the workings of the Chinese military (China Internet Information Center, 2007). The State Council Information Office issued a white paper on China's national defense in 2006 at a press conference on December 29 (State Council Information Office, 2007). The document, composed of 10 parts, summarizes the country's national-defense policy and the administration system, logistical support, scientific research, and international cooperation for national defense. In it, China proclaims that it will:

> take the scientific development outlook as an important guiding principle for the building of national defense and military affairs, vigorously advance the revolution in military affairs with Chinese features, and strive to realize an all-round, coordinated and sustainable development in our country's national defense and military capabilities.

Elsewhere, the white paper states that:

> keeping in mind the future informationized battlefield, the PLA [People's Liberation Army] closely follows the emerging trend of integrated joint operations, conducts integrated training in an innovative way, and actively explores training approaches for the internal integration of fighting units, systems integration of fighting elements and comprehensive integration of fighting systems.

The white paper also specifically mentions enhancing the performance of the armed forces with informationization, declaring that:

> the PLA pursues a strategy of strengthening itself by means of science and technology, and works to accelerate change in the generating mode of war fighting capabilities by drawing on scientific and technological advances . . . as well as defense-related science and technology, and strives to make major breakthroughs in some basic, pioneering and technological fields of strategic importance.

Although the paper does not directly mention specific details as to what technologies and science are to be used, it would not be too great a leap to suggest that the Chinese government is probably pursuing capability in cognitive neurosciences to enhance its national defense.

Several internationally accepted documents guide the ethical treatment of human participants in biomedical research. The most authoritative document is the WMA DoH, which is cited most often in the international literature and with which researchers across the globe at least claim to be in compliance. Although the international community largely accepts and respects the DoH, data on individual states' compliance are not available. The 1948 Universal Declaration of Human Rights in principle has global authority, but it is not invoked as often in the context of human-subjects research, although it does contain clear language about the ethical treatment of human subjects. In a legal context, such as during international tribunals, it is compelling. The oldest document, the 1947 Nuremberg Code, is not often cited directly as a reference document but has served as the foundation of other guiding documents, including the federal regulations in the United States. More recently, CIOMS issued the *International Ethical Guidelines for Biomedical Research Involving Human Subjects* (Council for International Organizations of Medical Sciences, 2002). Those guidelines are very detailed, practical, and sensitive to cultural differences between nations, but they may not have the same prominence as the DoH. In addition to those primary instruments, other national and international documents offer more specific guidance on separate subjects in biomedical research (for example, clinical trials and drug development).

The various guidelines agree on some main beliefs: that prior ethical review of research is required, that research must be justifiable and contribute to the well-being of society in general, that risk-benefit ratios must be reasonable, that informed consent or voluntariness is needed, that privacy a right, that data must be reported accurately, and that inappropriate behavior must be reported.

Individual nations may have their own ethical rules and regulations in addition to the international documents. For two nations in particular, Iran and China, we researched the existence and scope of such documents and the existence of evidence of research activity in cognitive neuroscience and biotechnology, specifically for military uses. Iran has detailed codes of medical ethics and biomedical research that have been officially ratified, and international documents have also been formally endorsed. There is some evidence that academic researchers may be developing capacity in neuroscience, especially in nanobiotechnology. What that implies for potential human or military uses and for compliance with ethical regulations is extremely difficult to assess.

China also claims to comply with the international instruments guiding research ethics. Although there has been considerable discussion in China about improved and more comprehensive guidelines for biomedical research with human subjects, no new documents have been ratified recently by the government. The Chinese government did, however, recently publish its goals for strengthening national defense, including the use of technological innovations and scientific breakthroughs to enhance the military (Cao, 2006; Simon, 2007).

From those findings, it follows that more investigation and insight are necessary regarding the compliance of several nations, including Iran and China, with international research-ethics directives and regarding their endeavors in biotechnologies, such as technologies related to cognitive neuroscience.

If studies are not submitted for publication or if applications for intellectual-property protection are not filed, there is no guarantee that they will come to the attention of the scientific community or of legal and regulatory authorities. The system for ensuring the ethics of human-research trials relies on a combination of international guidelines, various national regulatory systems, well-managed research institutions, and investigator self-reporting. To judge by long historical experience, system breakdowns are all too common. Therefore, the intelligence community's understanding of developments in this field cannot simply rely on current arrangements for the regulation of human research, nor can the international community be assured that human experiments that are exploitative and conducted for nefarious purposes are not taking place.

REFERENCES

Cao, Cong, Richard P. Suttmeier, and Denis Fred Simon. 2006. China's 15-year science and technology plan. *Physics Today* 59(12):38-43.
China Internet Information Center. 2007. Official Web site of the Chinese Government. State Council Information Office and the China International Publishing Group in Beijing, December 5, 2007.
Council for International Organizations of Medical Sciences. 2002. *International Ethical Guidelines for Biomedical Research Involving Human Subjects*. Geneva, Switzerland, November 2002. Available from http://www.cioms.ch/guidelines_nov_2002_blurb.htm. Last accessed June 8, 2008.

Hoge, Warren. 2007. Iran's president vows to ignore U.N. measures. *New York Times*. September 26, 2007. Available from http://www.nytimes.com/2007/09/26/world/26nations.html. Last accessed March 28, 2008.

Jahanshahi, Mohsen. 2005. Nanobiotechnology. Paper read at BINASIA-Iran National Workshop, November 8-9, 2005, Tehran, Iran.

Jia, Hepeng. 2006. China to release tougher rules for research ethics. *Science Development Network*, August 14. Available from http://www.scidev.net/News/index.cfm?fuseaction=readnews&itemid=3045&language=1.

Larijani, Bagher, and Farzaneh Zahedi. 2007. Medical ethics activities and plans in Iran at a glance. *Iranian Journal of Allergy, Asthma, and Immunology* 6(Suppl 5):1-4.

Renzong, Qui. 2007. China taking the right steps in bioethics. *Science Development Network*, May 18, 2007. Available from http://www.scidev.net/dossiers/index.cfm?fuseaction=dossierreaditem&dossier=5&type=3&itemid=611&language=1.

State Council Information Office. 2007. China's National Defense in 2006. Section 8, Science, Technology and Industry for National Defense. People's Republic of China, December 29, 2006. Available from http://www.china.org.cn/english/Books&Magazines/194419.htm#8.

United Nations. 1948. Universal Declaration of Human Rights. Adopted and proclaimed by General Assembly Resolution 217 A (III) of 10 December 1948. Palais de Chaillot, Paris, December 1948. Available from http://www.un.org/Overview/rights.html.

United Nations. 1966a. International Covenant on Civil and Political Rights. Adopted and opened for signature, ratification, and accession by General Assembly Resolution 2200A (XXI) of December 16, 1966. Entry into force March 23, 1976. Available from http://www.unhchr.ch/html/menu3/b/a_ccpr.htm.

United Nations. 1966b. International Covenant on Economic, Social and Cultural Rights. Adopted and opened for signature, ratification, and accession by General Assembly Resolution 2200A (XXI) of December 16, 1966. Entry into force January 3, 1976. Available from http://www.unhchr.ch/html/menu3/b/a_cescr.htm.

United Nations. 1979. Convention on the Elimination of All Forms of Discrimination Against Women. Adopted and opened for signature, ratification, and accession by General Assembly Resolution 34/180 of December 18, 1979. Entry into force September 3, 1981. Available from http://www.unhchr.ch/html/menu3/b/e1cedaw.htm.

United Nations. 1989. Convention on the Rights of the Child. Adopted and opened for signature, ratification, and accession by General Assembly Resolution 44/25 of November 20, 1989. Entry into force September 2, 1990. Available from http://www.unhchr.ch/html/menu3/b/k2crc.htm.

Williams, John R. 2005. Medical ethics in contemporary clinical practice. *Journal of the Chinese Medical Association* 68(11):495-499.

World Medical Association. 1964. Declaration of Helsinki: Ethical Principles for Medical Research Involving Human Subjects. Adopted by the 18th World Medical Association General Assembly. Helsinki, Finland, June 1964. Available from http://www.wma.net/e/policy/b3.htm.

Unpublished

Simon, Denis F. 2007. "China's Emerging Innovation Trajectory: The Competitive Implications." Presentation to the committee on August 15, 2007.

Appendix F

True and False Memories as an Illustrative Case of the Difficulty of Developing Accurate and Practical Neurophysiological Indexes of Psychological States

An important issue for cognitive neuroscientists concerns efforts to determine whether a person is reporting a true experience or one that is false but believed. In the last decade, there have been innumerable research efforts designed to distinguish true from false memories. Earlier work examining behavioral differences between true and false memories revealed that group differences were sometimes found (for example, more sensory details in true-memory reports) (Schooler et al., 1986). However, the statistical group differences did not enable reliable classification of any particular memory report as to its authenticity.

Some work with neuroimaging has attempted to locate differences in the brain that might reveal something about true and false memories. The goal of much of the work has been to demonstrate that true and false memories have different neural signatures (Curran et al., 2001; Fabiani et al., 2000; Miller et al., 2001). The allure of such research has been so great that considerable effort is likely to be devoted in the future to the neurophysiology of false memory. Despite some progress, we are far from being able to use neuroimaging techniques to tell us about the veracity of *particular* memories, because the reported findings are based on group averages. A group of true memories might show more activity in the visual cortex, whereas a group of false memories might show more activity in the auditory cortex. Group averages do not allow us to focus on an individual memory and to discern reliably whether it is true or false. Another potential problem with neuroimaging work on false memory is that such studies typically involve memory for words recently learned, and the few studies that have used this procedure have yielded inconsistent results. The methodological constraints of neuroimaging tools such as functional magnetic resonance imaging (fMRI) and event-related potentials make it difficult to study rich false memories.

A notable exception can be found in the work of Okado and Stark (2005), who examined true and false memories in the context of a misinformation experiment and thus studied richer false memories. Misinformation studies show how readily memory can become skewed when people are fed misinformation (Loftus, 2005). A typical misinformation study uses a simple three-stage procedure: subjects see a complex event, such as a simulated automobile accident; half the subjects receive misleading information about the accident, and the other half get no misinformation; and finally, all subjects try to remember the original accident. In one study that used that procedure, subjects saw an accident, and some of them later received misinformation about the traffic sign at the intersection in question. The misled subjects got the false suggestion that the stop sign that they had actually seen was a yield sign. When asked later what kind of traffic sign they remembered seeing, those who had been given the false suggestion tended to adopt it as their memory and claimed to have seen a yield sign. Hundreds of similar studies show that misinformation can change a person's recollection in predictable ways.

In an fMRI study that compared true memories with false memories created by misinformation, some group differences emerged (Okado et al., 2006). For example, the true-memory reports were associated with greater activation in the visual cortex, whereas the false-memory reports were associated with greater activation in the auditory cortex. However, the overwhelming impression from the research is that true and false memories are activating similar portions of the brain and that a particular memory cannot be reliably classified as true or false.

Richard McNally and his collaborators (McNally, 2003) studied people who had very rich, although likely false, memories of alien abduction have been studied. One study explored whether people who believe they have been abducted exhibit heightened physiological reactivity (heart rate and skin conductance) that occurs commonly in patients who have posttraumatic stress disorder (PTSD) when they think about their traumas. The "abductees" studied had experienced apparent sleep paralysis and hypnopompic hallucinations, which are vivid dreamlike hallucinations that occur as one is waking up, such as seeing figures hovering near their beds. Most had recovered memories with such techniques as guided imagery and hypnosis. Some of the recovered memories involved sexual intercourse with aliens or having sperm extracted for breeding purposes. Their physiological reactions were similar to those seen in PTSD patients who listen to audiotaped scripts of their traumas. Thus, expressed emotion is no guarantee that a memory is true.

There is a further concern in the true-memory–false-memory distinction: In many of the real-world cases, there have been attempts to get people to remember, to discuss their memories, to imagine details, and so on. Those very attempts can increase the detail and vividness of false memories—the very characteristics that lead (or rather mislead) people to believe that the memories are real.

REFERENCES

Curran, Tim, Daniel L. Schacter, Marcia K. Johnson, and Ruth Spinks. 2001. Brain potentials reflect behavioral differences in true and false recognition. *Journal of Cognitive Neuroscience* 13(2):201-216.

Fabiani, Monica, Michael A. Stadler, and Peter M. Wessels. 2000. True but not false memories produce a sensory signature in human lateralized brain potentials. *Journal of Cognitive Neuroscience* 12(6):941-949.

Loftus, Elizabeth F. 2005. Planting misinformation in the human mind: A 30-year investigation of the malleability of memory. *Learning and Memory* 12(4):361-366.

McNally, Richard J. 2003. *Remembering Trauma.* Cambridge, MA: Harvard University Press.

Miller, Antoinette R., Christopher Baratta, Christine Wynveen, and J. Peter Rosenfeld. 2001. P300 latency, but not amplitude or topography, distinguishes between true and false recognition. *Journal of Experimental Psychology: Learning, Memory, and Cognition* 27(2):354-361.

Okado, Yoko, Elizabeth Loftus, and Craig E.L. Stark. 2006. Imaging the reconstruction of true and false memories through sensory reactivation. Paper read at 13th Annual Cognitive Neuroscience Society Meeting, April 8-11, 2006, San Francisco, CA.

Okado, Yoko, and Craig E.L. Stark. 2005. Neural activity during encoding predicts false memories created by misinformation. *Learning and Memory* 12(1):3-11.

Schooler, Jonathan W., Delia Gerhard, and Elizabeth Loftus. 1986. Qualities of the unreal. *Journal of Experimental Psychology: Learning, Memory, and Cognition* 12(2):171-181.